The therapeutic procedures in this book are based on the training, personal experiences, and research of the author. Because each person and situation is unique, the author and publisher urge the reader to check with a qualified health professional before using any procedure where there is any question to appropriateness.

The publisher does not advocate the use of any particular diet or health program, but believes the information presented in this book should be available to the public.

Because there is always some risk involved, the author and publisher are not responsible for any adverse effects or consequences resulting from the use of any of the suggestions, preparations, or procedures in this book. Please do not use the book if you are unwilling to assume the risk. Feel free to consult with a physician or other qualified health professional.

OVERCOMING FIBROMYALGIA!
A Guide for Recovery

Written by
MARY MOELLER, LPN, TFH

TABLE OF CONTENTS

Acknowledgments

During these past numbers of years many people have provided me with the love, support and kindness that has been essential in helping me to continue my work. I would like to take this opportunity to thank these people.

I would like to begin first with Karl, my husband, for his love, friendship and support. It was his love and support that has given me the encouragement to continue my work in helping and supporting others who suffer with this devastating health issue. Karl's love kept me going during those dark years when others questioned the validity of my pain and symptoms. I thank God every day for Karl, my best friend and life-long love.

A special thank you also goes to Dr. Randy Dierenfield who first believed that there was hope of me feeling well again. Dr. Dierenfield's gentle guidance, encouragement and acupuncture treatments helped to lead me out of the depths of fibromyalgia and back to health. Also, thank you for all of the acupuncture treatments for Kelly to help aid in her recovery.

Thank you also to Kelly, my daughter, for following my lead when, at the age of 7, she came down with fms/cfs. Being the wonderful daughter she is, she dutifully made the changes in her diet, which ultimately reversed her symptoms.

Without the foresight and computer expertise of my son, Simon, this book and my work would not have been possible. While in junior high school, Simon designed the exercise pictures, and built a computer for me to begin my work. He also, because of his computer knowledge, talked Karl and I into buying a laptop computer, which we didn't feel we could afford at the time, but which has become the main tool used in my training courses and speaking engagements. The laptop made it possible for me to take my work to those who suffer as well as to those who would aspire to learn more about helping others with fibromyalgia and chronic fatigue.

Once our laptop was purchased, another very important person came into my life. Robert Trottman was intrumental in the design and construction of my fibromyalgia presentation. After being turned down by numerous others, Robert offered to help teach me how to build a PowerPoint presentation. He worked with me for months to create the presentation which ultimately became the basis for all the training presentations I do. Thank you, Robert, for lovingly giving of your time and energies to help me and to help fibromyalgia sufferers everywhere.

Thank you to Dr. William Shaw for his research in yeast and yeast related health issues. And, for his friendship and mentoring. Thank you also for providing very important information for this book about systemic yeast.

A big thank you to Dr. William Crook for his friendship and support. We all owe a great deal to Dr. Crook for his unending crusade to educate the world about yeast related health problems. Thank you also for allowing me to use the Candida Questionnaire from your book <u>Tired-So-Tired!</u>

Finally, I would like to thank Amanda Stever for editing this book. Without her help, I would have never made it. She was "a doll" to work with and did a great job!

Introduction

For those of us with fibromyalgia (FMS), life as we once knew it has changed dramatically. We know and understand all too well the symptoms and complaints we share as well as the lifestyle changes that have taken place since the onset of our symptoms. For me the symptoms started when I was in the seventh grade, long before the term "fibromyalgia" was in my physician's vocabulary. As with many other sufferers, my symptoms seemed to come on gradually, eventually consuming every part of my being. But, despite the painful control it had on my life, it wasn't until my daughter was diagnosed with FMS that I became serious about trying to combat the effects of this illness.

Many mornings, upon waking, I had mentioned to my husband that I didn't know if life was worth living if I had to live the rest of it in the extreme pain and with the overwhelming symptoms of fibromyalgia. Perhaps what was even more disturbing was to imagine my then 8-year-old daughter possibly developing those same feelings. So, with my daughter's and my own well being as a motivator, I set out on a long, challenging, and yes, rewarding journey to wellness. Together we accomplished something our doctors had told us could not be done: We reversed our symptoms!

Today my daughter and I share predominately symptom free, healthful lives. I am now able to do much more than I was able to do at 30 years of age and I feel great. My daughter, now an active and normal teenager, has the ability to enjoy life as fully as any other teenager. It was not easy, there were no magic pills to take to make the symptoms go away. We simply had to decide which we wanted most; to be, sick and confined to a life of pain and suffering or to be well and enjoy life to the fullest. This is not an illness that we can give to our doctors and expect to receive a "magic pill" which takes our symptoms away. Rather, it is an illness that requires us to look into the deepest canyons of our very being to decide what we truly value in life. There are many of us who have reversed the symptoms of fibromyalgia and chronic fatigue syndrome. It was not by chance that we were able to do this, rather by conscious choice and hard work.

In pondering the many changes that I have made in my life since making the decision to work towards becoming healthy again, I began thinking about those people who had helped me. One of the many people who helped form the mental picture of whom I would become was Dr. Wayne W. Dyer. In his book <u>Wisdom of the Ages</u>, Dr. Dyer discusses the dream state and allowing our dreams to become a part of our lives. Most everything we humans have accomplished began as a simple dream. A famous musician, Yanni, also talks about the ability of our minds to dream and through dreaming, create reality. Why then, can't our dreams of becoming healthy again become reality? Before we accomplish anything in our lives, it first begins as a dream. The home you now live in at one time was a dream in your mind. You may have chosen your living space for different reasons, but the basic dream of having a roof over your head was only in your mind until you found that home. Chairs to sit on and a stove on which to cook your food were at one time dreams in someone's mind. Maybe you are working at a job, or you have a family that you once dreamed of. Why not begin dreaming and seeing yourself as a whole, healthy person? Imagine having the energy to play a game of tennis, ride a bike, keep your house clean, go to a party. Or, your dream may be to comfortably cradle your newborn baby or grandchild. You can do it!

Once the dream of feeling well has become a part of you, it becomes necessary to begin taking steps to help bring about that dream. During our healing process, my daughter Kelly and I learned to change our lifestyle from one which included making poor health decisions to one of listening to our bodies and allowing our bodies to tell us what they needed to become and remain healthy. We learned to take time each day for play along with taking time to become quiet, to sit and just "be".

We realized that we had the rest of our lives to feel well, so we began to see this as a dream that would last a lifetime. This meant to begin working towards our dream each and every day, one day at a time. My dream was to feel completely well within a year and that goal was met in about that amount of time. You too can hold the dream of feeling well again. Set a goal which includes something you love to do but can no longer do because of this illness. Begin working towards that goal (dream.) As time passes, you will notice that each week you are doing more and feeling better. While weeks turn into months, each month you will notice small, yet wonderful, improvements as your body begins to return to a healthful state. Know you can feel well again. Healing must begin in your mind.

This book has been written to serve as a daily guide for you to follow, with each small step leading you to a new, healthier life. The style used is one of gentle guidance and support, so you will not feel like you are all alone in your journey. It is written very simply to help move you forward, even though you may have problems with memory and cognitive thinking. It is written for you, the sufferer, not academics or doctors. I have been where you are now and through this book, will guide you through each step, which I made to reclaim my life and health!

On those days in which you wonder if the work you are doing to feel well is worth the effort, stop for a quiet moment to remember your dream. It is worth every effort you are making. You will find life has so much more to offer when you are healthy and well. Remember, dream, then set goals that move you towards your dream. You can do it! I believe in you!

The Healing Process

After three months, Jan, a client I was working with, was feeling she had not gained anything from the program. She felt she had made the changes we had talked about, including that which was expected of her from the exercise program. She had become very frustrated and was about to give up. In looking back through our records and comparing her health evaluations, we found that she was now staying out of bed ten hours a day instead of the three hours she had when she first started the program. And she was now exercising between 30 and 60 minutes each day. A short three months before this time she was unable to exercise due to the extreme fatigue and pain. As she began to think about changes in her other symptoms it became obvious to her that there had been some significant improvements in her health. I reminded Jan about the conversation we had on the day she began working towards regaining her health. At that time I told her that the healing process is gradual and it is difficult to see changes from day to day. Rather, we need to look at increments of weeks or even months to compare and denote our progress. Many of the professionals I worked with as I was on my road to recovery had to remind me that I did not become sick overnight so it was not likely that I would become well overnight either. Often it takes months or even years to acquire the symptoms of FMS, so it may take some time for the body to heal. And unfortunately, even for those who have symptoms which appeared shortly after some physical or emotional trauma the symptoms take a period of time to go away. When Jan understood this, she was ready to continue to move forward, confidant that she was in fact, experiencing a very real and measurable journey to wellness.

In learning more about the human body and what it takes to become healthy, understand that it may take up to a year for an organ to restore itself. And some organs, such as the liver and brain, may take even longer. To better understand how this restorative process works, let's look at a severe sunburn. We all know that after spending a period of time in the sun, the skin turns brown or burns. After a week or two the burned layer will peal from the body. The burned, unhealthy cells have been replaced with new, healthy cells. When the process is complete, the old skin flakes off leaving behind healthy, new skin.

Revitalizing the organs of the body works in much the same way. Cells in our organs are constantly being replaced with new cells. If our body is not getting proper nutrition to create new cells which are healthy, the old cells may be replaced with unhealthy new cells, creating a weakened organ. Understanding this concept, my goal was to give my body what it needed to build healthy cells to replace the unhealthy cells. It became obvious that if the organs of my body were healthy, my body as a whole would be healthy also.

As many of my symptoms began to diminish, my memory and cognitive thinking processes seemed to be improving at a much slower rate. In fact, my problems with memory and cognitive thinking were the last to go away. I was beginning to fear that the memory lapses and inability to comprehend and properly utilize information would always be with me. Finally, after about eleven months, I noticed some improvement. I was reading the local newspaper when I noticed that I was not having any problem remembering what I was reading. Improvement had been so gradual that I had not noticed it.

There are many theories about the causes of fibromyalgia and chronic fatigue syndrome. Numerous people who suffer from this illness have studied the scientific literature to learn as much as possible so they can better understand how this illness could have extracted such a toll on their lives. And there is a lot to study. A new theory seems to cross my desk every six months or so. A few of the theories look at neurochemical disorders or distorted pain perception while other studies look at improper serotonin levels or substance P factors. Some studies have looked at the possibility of the body's inability to excrete phosphates efficiently while still another possibility, metabolic dysfunction, constitutes a problem of utilizing or eliminating certain substances in the body. And though a genetic link has still not been proven, we know that fibromyalgia and chronic fatigue syndrome tends to run in families. Still another theory is that ACTH, which is a hormone that enables the proper function of the adrenal gland, may be affected by the common flu. This then begins the downhill spiral of health leading to symptoms of FMS and CFS.

What we do know is that fibromyalgia and chronic fatigue syndrome affects the immune system, and that some doctors consider it to be an autoimmune problem. We also know that systemic yeast problems have the ability to cause or create many of the symptoms associated with FMS and CFS and that when the yeast has been eliminated, the multitude of symptoms will usually go away too.

Let me give you an example of how this can work. A while back, a lady whose husband had been diagnosed with chronic fatigue syndrome contacted me. His health was spiraling downward very quickly. And he was contemplating quitting his job, as it was becoming almost impossible for him to muster the energy to fight the pain and extreme fatigue during his workday. After meeting with them in my office, I referred him to a doctor who found that he had a systemic yeast problem. We changed his diet and started him on a customized exercise program. At the same time we began to aggressively go after his yeast problem with a dietary supplement. In addition, a good vitamin and mineral supplement program was designed and implemented. Within four weeks his energy was returning, pain was lessening and his sleep was beginning to deepen. Within three months he was almost completely symptom free and was sleeping deeply for seven to eight hours each night. By that time he had more energy and was feeling so much better than his "healthy" wife that she decided to make some changes in her life so she would be able to keep up with him.

Another lady, after making the lifestyle changes outlined in my first book, Fibromyalgia Cookbook, and treating her yeast overgrowth problem, found that she was able to once again drive her car to the store to purchase her own groceries. And she was able to exercise and do light yard work for periods lasting between one to three hours. Of course, as she continued to give her body what it needed to restore itself to health, her symptoms became even less of a factor in her life.

To reverse symptoms it was very important to begin working towards building a healthier body and immune system. Most doctors who are successfully treating fibromyalgia work towards treating causes, rather than symptoms. In treating causes, many of these doctors are looking to the immune system for answers in helping patients regain optimum health. As we learn more about the immune system, we find that it plays an important role in maintaining health. Research has found that an unhealthy immune system may be instrumental in creating the downhill slides known as fibromyalgia and chronic fatigue syndrome. In looking at the role of the immune system, we must understand that it encompasses the entire body. In better understanding the immune system, we find when one area of the body is stressed, it may put stress on another area of the body. In his book, The Downhill Syndrome, Pavel Yutsis, M.D., discusses the numerous stresses on our immune system. A few of these stresses may include eating too many processed foods, yeast infections and toxic agents such as pesticides and insecticides.

When we consider that an immune system problem can bring about a multitude of the symptoms of FMS and CFS, it becomes necessary to look at ways to help it become strong again. When I began my journey toward health, my focus turned from applying symptomatic treatment, to practicing holistic treatment by giving my body everything it needed to improve and heal. With a background in nursing, my original focus was on treating symptoms rather than causes. While operating under that philosophy my health continued to spiral downward. But, what I found after a few weeks looking at the problem wholelistically shocked me. As my immune system began to respond and become stronger, the symptoms began to lessen and my sleep deepened. In fact today, many of my clients find that after making a just few dietary changes, their sleep begins to deepen and they awake feeling more rested. Since sleep depravation can cause symptoms which mimic those of FMS and CFS, the better your sleep the more likely it is that your body will be able to rebuild itself. But, beyond sleep, all symptoms improve considerably when the body is treated as a whole.

My daughter and I succeeded in regaining our health without the aid of prescription medication. However, this program is in no way meant to replace your medical treatment, or regular trips to your physician. Over time, while continuing consultations with your physician, you may find trips to the doctor will become less frequent. And as your need for medications becomes less, your doctor can help work you off of them.

Many times I meet fibromyalgia sufferers who have read every book available on FMS and CFS. Their comment is "I know all there is to know about fibromyalgia and nothing works, I am still not better." Knowing everything is not the same as putting to use what you have learned. Reversing the symptoms does not come from cerebral knowledge as much as it comes from applied knowledge. A house is not built through the dream itself, or from the knowledge of how to build it. It is built through hard, "hands on" work. Become a person who is willing to do the work it takes to feel better. A body ridden with fibromyalgia will have a difficult time becoming healthy if the knowledge its' brain has is not utilized. It is only through making the changes and working towards building a healthy body that the healing process will be given a chance to become a reality.

Understanding the Process of Reversing Fibromyalgia

During the past few years of working with thousands of fibromyalgia and chronic fatigue sufferers, it has become obvious to me that this illness can strike rather abruptly. When it does it is generally associated with a traumatic incident. In his book, Reversing Fibromyalgia, Dr. Joe Elrod talks about the effects of emotional or physical trauma when combined with a poor diet, lack of exercise and vitamin deficiencies. The result of this combination, according to Dr. Elrod, is that trauma can serve as a catalyst for fibromyalgia if the body's immune system has already been compromised through years of living an unhealthy lifestyle. The weakened immune system may then perpetuate the symptoms of fibromyalgia.

To reverse FMS and CFS then, whether triggered by a trauma, or if it was manifested over a period of years, the common need is to strengthen the immune system. That is the primary purpose of this book. I will walk with you through three months of results oriented, lifestyle changes. These changes encompass our diets, exercise and sleep habits. You will see the results in your own body.

One can expect anywhere from one to three months of work on these changes before any positive effects can be seen in the symptoms.

Reversing the symptoms of FMS and CFS will not happen overnight, because remember, we all spent years unknowingly working towards acquiring it.

Beginning the Healing Process

Many times our first thought in finding a solution to our pain or sleeplessness is to go to the drugstore to find a pill which will alleviate the symptoms. That solution may work, although, I have found that for Kelly and myself, those solutions have not been as effective as the remedies we can find in our own gardens or in health food stores. And it is always important for me to remember that the way to permanently alleviate the problem is to get rid of the underlying cause. Otherwise we are just putting a bandage on the symptoms.

My goal from the beginning was and is to change what I need to improve within my life to create a healthy body. In doing that, the symptoms automatically take care of themselves. This should also become a life long, maintenance program. If we go back to our old habits once we feel better, the symptoms will recur as our bodies begin to once again struggle to remain healthy.

It is very important to follow this book on a daily basis to feel better. Take it with you as your daily planner so you will be able to keep accurate records. Keeping it near your side will help you avoid some of the "no-no's" which could throw you off track, along with giving you encouragement to keep trying. If you slip periodically, that is okay. Start again the next day. Remember, you did not get this illness overnight, it may take awhile to feel better, so if you slip up, you always have tomorrow to begin again. This may be one of the toughest challenges you will ever have to overcome. I will try to help, so that together we can do it. And take some comfort in knowing that thousands of others have successfully been down the same road which you are taking your first steps on today. You will be so happy you did. And I will be happy for you!

The daily guide portion of this book is designed to help you make the lifestyle changes necessary to begin the healing process. It covers the first 90 days, and works the sufferer into a very gradual, yet comprehensive pattern of healthy living. Once you have covered approximately three months of lifestyle changes, you will have what you need to continue your journey to feeling and keeping healthy.

There is a section in the back of the book which covers natural remedies for pain control, sleep disturbances, muscle relaxation and muscle stretching exercises. Refer to this section whenever you need helpful hints in these areas. And remember, always consult with your physician or health professional before embarking on this, or any other journey to health!

I chose a more natural means to control our symptoms since we found that if pills helped one problem, they also seemed to create another. For Kelly and myself, I feel the natural forms of sleep enhancers and pain control are much more effective. Experiment on your own and take note of what your body is telling you as far as how the remedy is affecting it. If you notice a "different" or uncomfortable feeling from taking something, chances are you should try something else. This is where quiet time each day comes in. As a person quiets themselves and their mind, a whole new realm of intuitive feelings can come about, along with a new sense of serenity about your condition.

Systemic Yeast and Fibromyalgia

A common thread, systemic yeast overgrowth, seems to be widely overlooked and scoffed at by many medical professionals. However, those who are successfully helping their fibromyalgia and chronic fatigue patients back to full health recognize the validity of systemic yeast and its role in causing symptoms common to this illness.

In looking at the causes of systemic yeast in the human body, we find many factors may lead to this very real health problem. According to Dr. William Crook, author of numerous books on systemic yeast, antibiotics, birth control pills, tetracycline's and other commonly used medications may begin an avalanche of health issues which begin with a systemic yeast overgrowth. Usage of these and many other drugs creates an imbalance in normal flora within the body allowing an overgrowth of "bad" yeast. As this process continues, more and more symptoms common to fibromyalgia and chronic fatigue begin to appear.

Some researchers believe systemic yeast issues may be present in a large percentage of people who suffer with fibromyalgia and chronic fatigue syndrome. Doctors have related systemic yeast problems in difficult to treat patients with symptoms of fatigue, depression, and vaginal discomfort since the 1960's.

Although treatment of systemic yeast problems may seem fairly simple, it can be difficult. Simple dietary changes, such as removal of wheat based breads, processed foods, dairy products, sugars and sugar substitutes are necessary to keep from feeding the yeast. Introducing a pro and pre-biotic to kill off bad yeast and replace it with a balance of good yeast is the next step. It is also very important to get proper exercise and practice a well-rounded nutritional program to help the body regenerate healthy cells which replace old cells as they die and to rid the body of the toxins which are released when the bad yeast dies off.

In general, when following the protocol in this book, and when using a pro and pre biotic to aid in ridding the body of systemic yeast, the first "die-off" may occur within three to six weeks after beginning the program. Before the initial die-off occurs, one may notice a craving for sugar, sweets, breads or salty foods. Once this occurs, within approximately three to five days, what seems to be a relapse will occur. This happens, in part, from the toxins released from the yeast as it dies. It is important to continue drinking plenty of water, and exercising, if possible. Sweating during this process is also helpful in ridding the body of toxins left behind from the yeast that has died. According to Dr. Jeannie Driscoe of the University of Kansas Medical Center, using Alka Seltzer Gold with both soluble and insoluble fiber during this period may be helpful in lessening the symptoms. This die-off period may last from three days up to two weeks. It is very important to continue the diet and nutritional program during this period. Once a die-off has occurred and the toxins have been released from the body, one generally feels noticeably better. Sleep is generally much deeper and longer, irritable bowel syndrome is improved, indigestion generally dissipates, pain is decreased, and many of other symptoms are either greatly lessened or have subsided.

Eating Habits

Eating has become a passion for Americans. Almost everything we do revolves around eating. Generally, the foods available for us are not healthy. Holiday and party tables are laden with sweets, fats, and carbonation. Those foods that may resemble something healthy many times are covered with tasteful coatings containing preservatives, salts or sugars. Wherever we turn, food is in front of us, and it usually is not in a form that is nutritious for the body. We eat because we are happy. We eat because we are sad. We eat to celebrate or to mourn. Food becomes our friend. And many times when our health begins to fail, food seems to be the one thing in life which we can still enjoy.

Despite watching their diets and noticing improvement in their health, many of my clients are tempted to go back to their old eating habits. Within days or even hours, they begin to feel badly again. For example, Carol, a client who had been on my program for nine months, had been feeling pretty good for a couple of months. Along came Easter, with all of its chocolate delights and dinners. Carol thought she had felt well long enough that it would not make a difference if she celebrated Easter in the manner she had been accustomed to in the past. That form of celebrating included several meals where large servings of fresh breads, candies and other "goodies" were consumed. Within two days after binging Carol lost energy and began to have pain and extreme cravings for sugars and sweets. When she called she was very frustrated.

She could not imagine that the foods she had eaten over that short week could create such havoc in her health. I explained to Carol that it may take up to fifteen months for every cell in the body to heal, and that if she had systemic yeast when she came to me nine months before, it could come back at any time if she began eating candies and breads. After our visit, she took those foods back out of her diet and within a couple of weeks she was feeling great! Today we laugh, together, about her "learning experience."

Most Americans run around tired and exhausted without relating their lack of energy to the foods they eat. We have become a very sick and tired society. We need to wake up and realize the fuel we put into our bodies determines how much energy we have. If I am short on sleep, eating only foods that are very high in nutrition, easily digested, and drinking plenty of water, can greatly reduce my fatigue. This is because my body's energy is not being drained by fighting to process heavy foods. My body is getting the nutrition it needs to function in a form that is easily digested. We would not put oil-laden fuel into an engine and expect it to function at optimum level. So why would we do it to our own bodies?

Well, you can not eat right without preparing it. "Cooking for recovery" does not need to be difficult or to take a long time. Sometimes the most difficult obstacle to overcome is our mental attitude toward cooking and eating healthy. Many times my clients are not sure they want or are ready to, give up highly processed and artificially flavor enhanced foods. But one does not have to sacrifice flavor. Interestingly, when we eat fresh or steamed foods combined with fresh herbs, the flavors are astonishing! And, if we remember to keep as close to nature as possible, meals can be a snap! A few fresh fruits, vegetables and a bean, chicken, turkey or fish entrée, and the meal is on the table. Those who have digestive disturbances from raw food may find lightly steaming foods to be beneficial. (Drinking a cup of ginger and/or peppermint tea may also help.)

Many FMS and CFS sufferers have an intolerance to red meats. This may, in part, be due to the antibiotics and other medications used in feed for livestock. Or it simply may be due to their body's inability to digest red meats. To determine if you are sensitive to any foods, including meats, take the food out of your diet for two weeks. Then have a meal with that particular food in it. If your system is somewhat intolerant of it, you will know almost immediately. Most common symptoms that may indicate sensitivities to a food are indigestion, bloating, gas and headaches. Another quick, easy way to determine if you are sensitive to a food is to take a simple pulse test. To do this, take your pulse before ingesting the food, then 20 minutes after ingesting the food and again one hour later. If the body is sensitive to a food, the pulse will rise on the second reading and go back to normal by the third reading.

As the body heals and becomes stronger, it is still important to continue your healthy eating habits as much as possible. "Cheating" for a meal here or there may not be an issue, although, when cheating becomes a regular occurrence, symptoms may begin to return. Remember, eating should be a source of energy as well as enjoyment. Learn how to create fun, interesting and flavorful foods which are also healthy.

As you begin to make healthy changes in foods prepared for parties and special occasions, you will find others appreciate the change also. One Christmas, I hosted an annual party for members of my church at my home. I was fairly new to the group, but Janice, the lady in charge of snacks, knew that I ate "health food." So she kindly informed me that she had brought a plate of fruits, vegetables and dips for me, and that the rest of the group would be munching on candies, cookies, brownies and coffee. As Janice and I visited, she told me sweets and coffee were the food and drink of choice with this group and so they were served at every meeting. I made a pot of mint tea for myself, offering it to anyone who was interested, but knowing that, as usual, I would be happily enjoying it and my "health food" alone. After the party was over and most everyone was gone Janice and I made an interesting discovery. All of the fruits and vegetables were gone, and in the course of the evening, I had made three pots of mint tea to quench their thirsts. Only one brownie and one cookie had been eaten! We laughed as Janice packed her cookies and brownies up to take home to her family.

On another occasion, my family and I attended an "end of the school year" party held at our daughter's school. Each family was to bring a snack to share with the rest. I was astounded as I looked at the food spread on the thirty-foot long table. Chips, cookies and brownies covered the entire table, except for two dishes. These two dishes contained vegetables, with dip, and fruit, with dip. Before half of those attending the party were through the line, the fruits and vegetables were gone!

It is time to begin to rethink what we serve at celebrations. Are we providing foods that will help keep our friends healthy, or are we simply providing something to eat? Don't be shy in providing healthy choices for activities. Set an example. Like me, you may be surprised at how many people appreciate them!

Making healthy eating a habit should be a life long endeavor, not a short term goal. As you begin to feel better, look for ways to prepare healthful dishes you can share with others. It may surprise you how many others appreciate the healthy foods you have created.

Nutritional Supplementation

During the healing process and continuing through the present, taking vitamin and mineral supplementation has been imperative for me to become and remain healthy. When you begin taking vitamin and mineral supplementation it may take time to notice improvements in the way you feel. The reason is quite simple. It takes time for vitamins and minerals to build up in the body.

To better understand how this may work, consider the analogy of a car engine. If a car engine looses all of its' oil, it is necessary to initially pour more oil into the engine to fill it up than in ensuing oil additions. This is because the engine's reservoir is dry and needs to be brought up to a certain minimal level to be effective. If you were to only add a little at a time, the engine would labor against the resistance caused by friction. But, assuming the engine did not seize up before you added enough oil, eventually it would begin running smoothly. Like a car engine, our bodies must receive enough vitamins and minerals. And, like an engine, the sooner we build our reservoir to an effective level, the better off we will be.

I feel it is important to understand also that all vitamins are not created equal. Several of the supplements I tried seemed to have little or no effect, even after using them for months. Look for quality supplements that are backed by clinical studies on products selected at random from a company's consumer ready product. For example, anyone can site a study about the value of vitamin C, but does their product actually get the active component to where it needs to be in the body?

Most of us are aware that along with a healthy diet, additional supplementation is very important. But do we know why? Minerals, which contribute to high vitamin and mineral content in fruits and vegetables, simply are no longer in the soil. This absence of vitamins and minerals in the foods we eat can help contribute to many health problems. It may be necessary to supplement vitamin and minerals through nutritional supplements, as your body can not make most vitamins and minerals. But what are these health problems and what do vitamins and minerals really do? Looking at vitamin deficiencies and their symptoms may help to find some answers to these questions.

Vitamins, organic compounds, are indispensable to maintain appropriate body functions. Proper growth, health and reproduction depend upon vitamins. All vitamins play important roles in our health. Some vitamins are crucial for growth, while other vitamins are imperative for proper biological processes to take place in cells. Still others are essential for repair and maintenance of cells.

The human body cannot make most vitamins and minerals so they must be derived from foods or supplements. As mentioned above, studies now show our soils do not contain enough minerals to enable plants to contain the amount of vitamins and minerals they once did. Other changes (such as breeding for plant size, increased shelf life, size, color, and mechanized harvesting) may produce plants that are much lower in vitamins and minerals than in years gone by. And compounding the problem, our bodies are changing too. As our bodies grow older, poor digestion may slowly cause problems with the absorption and utilization of nutrients in foods. Over a period of time this situation can be instrumental in worsening the problem of vitamin deficiencies.

With all the above in mind, we are reminded of why we need supplementation. We know the general uses our bodies make of vitamins and minerals, however, in taking a closer look, we find there are more specific purposes for vitamins and minerals in the body.

In total there are thirteen vitamins. Those that are stored in the body's fat, also known as fat soluble, are vitamins A, D, K, and E. Those that are not stored in the body (water-soluble) are vitamin C, and the B vitamins. The B vitamins are B-1 (Thiamin), B-2 (Riboflavin), B-6 (Pantothenic Acid), B-12, folic acid and biotin. Their specific purposes are as follows:

Vitamin A is required for healthy vision and a strong immune system, supporting kidney and liver function, healthy skin, and normal wound healing. Too much vitamin A can cause adverse health problems. Symptoms of deficiencies might include small, hard bumps on the skin (goose or toad flesh), night blindness or weak eyesight. Vitamin A may be used in the treatment of the following disorders: renew aged skin and treatment of acne; mucous membrane, lung or intestinal epithelial cancers, low function of the thymus and thyroid gland.

Vitamin D is needed for the growth of healthy bones and teeth and in the assimilation of vitamin A.

Vitamin K helps to regulate normal blood clotting. Lower levels may contribute to suppression of the immune system. Requires a small amount of dietary fat in the small intestine to be absorbed.

Vitamin E is required for the formation of red blood cells, maintaining cell membranes and is an antioxidant. Deficiencies are not seen in humans except after prolonged periods of fat absorption.

Vitamin C is beneficial in healing wounds by keeping blood vessels strong. Additionally, it is beneficial in helping the body resist infections and regulating blood sugar along with supporting liver and kidney function. It also helps to keep the heart strong and it possibly can inhibit formation of cataracts, relieve allergies and support kidney and liver function. Symptoms of deficiencies may include dry scaly skin, pin point hemorrhages under the skin, break down of old scars, loosened teeth, muscle cramps, tender joints, swollen joints, bleeding gums, swollen legs and arms, depression and shortness of breath.

B Vitamins help in maintaining a healthy liver, kidneys, and nervous system. Furthermore, it contributes to proper growth and muscle tone, aids in carbohydrate, fat and protein metabolism and in the formation of antibodies. Other functions of the body, such as a healthy cardiovascular system, depend on the B vitamin folic acid, B6 and B12. Folic Acid is essential for blood formation, maintaining cells genetic code by providing normal growth and maintenance of all cells. Available through leafy green vegetables and nutritional supplementation, folic acid deficiencies may contribute to fatigue. Respiratory problems may be related to deficiencies in vitamins B1, B12 and B6. Other symptoms of B vitamin deficiencies may include mental confusion, muscle weakness, edema, loss of appetite, sensitivity to light, cracking in corners of the mouth, dermatitis, smooth tongue, numbing and tingling in fingers and toes, and pernicious anemia.

Minerals also play an important role in health and are fundamental in providing for the proper metabolism of carbohydrates, fat and protein. Minerals also help nerve impulses crucial for the functioning of the heart and muscles, and create proper bone growth. As the body does not manufacture minerals and it is difficult for an FM stressed body to utilize minerals from food, nutritional supplementation may be the best source. Let's take a look at some specific minerals.

Calcium is vital in the lifelong development and maintenance of healthy bones and teeth. It helps in preventing cancer, clotting blood, regulating blood pressure, producing enzymes and hormones, preventing heart disease, transporting nutrients across cell membranes, normal muscle contraction (including heartbeat), maintaining a healthy nervous system and keeping teeth strong.

Since magnesium and phosphorus help maintain health in every aspect of the body, deficiency of these minerals can affect any or all functions of the body.

Potassium, sodium and chloride (essential for the body to function efficiently) are in all body fluids which keep your PH balance stabilized and are essential in keeping muscles and nerves healthy. Chloride also aids in digestion.

Sulfur and chromium play yet another role in helping maintain health as they are both required in helping the body to regulate insulin.

We now know why supplementation of vitamins and minerals is so critical to our bodies. And it is perhaps even more important to fibromyalgia sufferers as studies show they are usually vitamin and mineral deficient. Poor diets, weakened digestive systems and foods grown in depleted soils may be an important piece to the puzzle of the causes of fibromyalgia and chronic fatigue syndrome. Could it be the hype about vitamins and minerals does have greater merit than many give it credit for?

Beginning Your Road to Health

The following instructions will help you get the most from this book. Please read them carefully before continuing. The guide in this book will help you eliminate the following foods from your diet: chocolate, carbonation, coffee, alcohol, white or wheat flours, sugars and processed foods. Since most of these foods contain little or no nutritional value and they may cause additional stress on the liver, it is important to eliminate them. This may be done over a period of time (90 Day Guide) or they may be taken out all at once (Cold Turkey). Whether cutting these foods out all at once, or working them out over a period of time, it is crucial to follow the exercise program for each day.

Cold Turkey: For some, eliminating the above foods all at one time is the best approach. For those who choose to go "cold turkey" use the chart immediately following the last Health Evaluation Form, (after Day 90) as a daily checklist of dietary instructions. Photocopy it and post it in some convenient place, such as on the refrigerator. Check items off daily as they are completed, consumed, or not consumed, as the case may be. This checklist will also serve as a daily reminder of those foods to stay away from.

Although, my experience has been that those who use the "cold turkey" approach heal quicker, this approach is not for everyone. Those who use this approach can expect to begin to crave some or all of these foods within a period of about three to four weeks after taking them out of their diet. This craving may last for a number of days. If one can make it through this period of time without eating the foods they are craving, the healing process will be much quicker. If, however, they do not successfully make it through the time of intense cravings, their healing time will, obviously, take longer. For this reason, I find that it is easier for most to follow the three-month daily guide. The cravings do not seem to be nearly as intense when eliminating these foods over a period of time.

Exercise: Exercise is one of the body's tools which it utilizes in eliminating toxins. As the body continues its healing process, it is very important to help with this process through proper exercise and drinking plenty of water. Whether following the three-month daily guide or eliminating all the bad foods at once, exercise remains a very important facet in healing.

Many times sufferers will feel worse after exercising. According to Dr. Joe Elrod, author of Reversing Fibromyagia, this may be due to nutritional deficiencies. If this is your situation, it may be helpful to get on a good, reputable, nutritional program for approximately two weeks before exercising. This gives the body time to replenish nutritional deficiencies before using muscles that are too deficient to function.

What To Expect While Using This Book and After The First Three Months

While using this program, you will experience hills and valleys. This is why filling out the Health Evaluation Form (HEF) is so important. It will help be your guide in knowing you are improving. In the beginning, one can expect to have more bad than good days, although, as time continues on, there will be equal amounts of good and bad days. Finally, within about three to four months, there should be more good than bad days.

As time goes on, for up to one year, symptoms should not be as dramatic in intensity, and eventually become very light, until they are finally gone. During the first few months, hang onto those "good" days. Continue seeing the good days in your mind, even as you are experiencing the "bad" days. The healing process takes time, just as it took time to prepare your body for being sick. You can do it!

Beginning the Program

You are now ready to begin your journey to better health. Remember, this may take some time. It took me almost a full year to feel well again. I did not see much improvement before three months, and after that the changes were still very gradual. You could take less or more time depending on your own body and how fast it is able to heal itself.

Many times when I was feeling very bad due to the fibromyalgia, it was difficult for me to comprehend the words I was trying to read. To make the instructions easier to follow, in much of the workbook, I have made it **simple and repetitive**. I hope this will make the workbook easier for you to follow also.

1. Before beginning the daily pages of the workbook, fill out the first Health Evaluation Form (HEF). Using numbers from 1-10, with 1 being the least frequency or intensity and 10 being the greatest frequency or intensity, record what your current condition is. In other words, if you felt great, you would record all 1's, and if you like death warmed over, you would record all 10's.
2. If you have purchased the audiotape **Overcoming Fibromyalgia and Chronic Fatigue Syndrome,** listen to it now. It will explain more about the symptoms you may be having and what your body may be trying to tell you through these symptoms. For example, why you may be waking up many times during the night, what may be causing the tender spots on your body and in general, why the changes in this book are necessary.

3. Familiarize yourself with the exercise program and read the chapters on Natural Sleep Aids and Natural Pain Aids in the back of the book.
4. Look at some of the recipes for ideas on preparing foods.
5. Take the candida test in the Candida questionaire and score sheet section.
6. Determine if you would like to follow the daily guide or make all of the lifestyle changes at one time. If you are making the changes all at one time, review the "Cold Turkey" section in the chapter entitled, "Beginning Your Road to Health." If you are not quite up to going "cold turkey," and most of us are not, then continue on to step seven.
7. Take a deep breath and begin with Day 1. Your life is about to change.

Candida Questionnaire
And Score Sheet

(Used with Permission, <u>Tired-So Tired!</u>, Dr. William Crook)

Section A: History

		Point Score
1.	Have you ever taken tetracyclines or other antibiotics for acne for one month (or longer)?	35
2.	Have you at any time in your life taken broad-spectrum antibiotics or other antibacterial medications for respiratory, urinary or other infections for two months or longer, or in shorter courses four or more times in a one-year period?	35
3.	Have you taken a broad-spectrum antibiotic drug-even in a single dose?	6
4.	Have you, at any time in your life, been bothered by persistent prostatitis, vaginitis or other problems affecting your reproductive organs?	25
5.	Are you bothered by memory or concentration problems-do you sometimes feel "spaced out"?	20
6.	Do you feel "sick all over" yet, in spite of visits to many different physicians, the causes haven't been found?	20
7.	Have you been pregnant...	
	Two or more times?	5
	One time?	3
8.	Have you taken birth control pills...	
	For more than two years?	15
	For six months to two years?	8
9.	Have you taken steroids orally, by injection or inhalation?	
	For more than two weeks?	15
	For two weeks or less?	6
10.	Does exposure to perfumes, insecticides, fabric shop odors and other chemicals provoke...	
	Moderate or severe symptoms?	20
	Mild symptoms?	5
11.	Does tobacco smoke really bother you?	10
12.	Are your symptoms worse on damp muggy days or in moldy places?	20
13.	Have you had athlete's foot, ringworm, "jock itch" or other chronic fungous infections of the skin or nails? Have such infections been...	
	Severe or persistent?	20
	Mild to moderate?	10
14.	Do you crave sugar?	10

TOTAL SCORE, Section A _____

Section B: Major Symptoms

For each of your symptoms, enter the appropriate figure in the Point Score column:

     If a symptom is occasional or mild.....................................3 points
     If a symptom is frequent and/or moderately severe..........6 points
     If a symptom is sever and/or disabling ....9 points

Add total score and record it at the end of this section.

		Point Score
1.	Fatigue or lethargy	___
2.	Feeling of being "drained"	___
3.	Depression or manic depression	___
4.	Numbness, burning or tingling	___
5.	Headache	___
6.	Muscle aches	___
7.	Muscle weakness or paralysis	___
8.	Pain and/or swelling in joints	___
9.	Abdominal pain	___
10.	Constipation and/or diarrhea	___
11.	Bloating, belching or intestinal gas	___
12.	Troublesome vaginal burning, itching or discharge	___
13.	Prostatitis	___
14.	Impotence	___
15.	Loss of sexual desire	___
16.	Endometriosis or infertility	___
17.	Cramps and/or other menstrual irregularities	___
18.	Premenstrual tension	___
19.	Attacks of anxiety or crying	___
20.	Cold hands or feet, low body temperature	___
21.	Hypothyroidism	___
22.	Shaking or irritable when hungry	___
23.	Cystitis or interstitial cystitis	___
	TOTAL SCORE, Section B	___

Section C: Other Symptoms

For each of your symptoms, enter the appropriate figure in the Point Score column:

     If a symptom is occasional or mild . . . . .1 point

     If a symptom is frequent and/or moderately severe . . . . .2 points

     If a symptom is severe and/or disabling . . . . .3 points

Add total score and record it at the end of this section.

	Point Score
1. Drowsiness, including inappropriate drowsiness	___
2. Irritability	___
3. Incoordination	___
4. Frequent mood swings	___
5. Insomnia	___
6. Dizziness/loss of balance	___
7. Pressure above ears... feeling of head swelling	___
8. Sinus problems...tenderness of cheekbones or forehead	___
9. Tendency to bruise easily	___
10. Eczema, itching eyes	___
11. Psoriasis	___
12. Chronic hives (urticaria)	___
13. Indigestion or heartburn	___
14. Sensitivity to milk, wheat, corn or other common foods	___
15. Mucus in stools	___
16. Rectal itching	___
17. Dry mouth or throat	___
18. Mouth rashes, including "white" tongue	___
19. Bad breath	___
20. Foot, hair or body odor not relieved by washing	___
21. Nasal congestion or postnasal drip	___
22. Nasal itching	___
23. Sore throat	___
24. Laryngitis, loss of voice	___
25. Cough or recurrent bronchitis	___
26. Pain or tightness in chest	___
27. Wheezing or shortness of breath	___
28. Urinary frequency or urgency	___
29. Burning on urination	___
30. Spots in front of eyes or erratic vision	___
31. Burning or tearing eyes	___
32. Recurrent infections or fluid in ears	___
33. Ear pain or deafness	___
TOTAL SCORE, Section C	___
Total Score, Section A	___
Total Score, Section B	___
GRAND TOTAL SCORE	___

The Grand Total Score will help you and your physician decide if your health problems are yeast-connected. Scores in women will run higher, as seven items in the questionnaire apply exclusively to women, while only two apply exclusively to men.

Yeast-connected health problems are almost certainly present in women with scores more than 180, and in men with scores more than 140.

Yeast-connected health problems are probably present in women with scores more than 120, and in men with scores more than 90.

Yeast-connected health problems are possibly present in women with scores more than 60, and in men with scores more than 40.

With scores of less than 60 in women and 40 in men, yeasts are less apt to cause health problems.

HEALTH EVALUATION FORM

Indicate in the column next to the symptoms which of the following conditions apply to you in terms of frequency and/or intensity using the numbers 1-10: With 1 indicating the least and 10 indicating the greatest intensity or frequency.

Low Energy	____	Often Feel Tired	____	Headaches	____
Dry/Itchy Skin	____	Dry or Itchy Scalp	____	Rashes or Eczema	____
Achy Joints	____	Muscle Cramps	____	Muscle Twitches	____
Bruising	____	Menstrual Cramps	____	Moody/PMS	____
Poor Concentration	____	Water Retention	____	Bowel Gas	____
Numbing/Tingling	____	Skin Burning	____	Dry Eyes	____
Weak Fingernails	____	Dry/Brittle Hair	____	Weak Muscles	____
Joint Pain	____	Foot Pain	____	TMJ Pain	____

Indigestion/Acid Reflux	____	Constipation and/or Diarrhea	____
Frequently Take Pain Killers	____	Difficulty Handling Stress	____
High/Low Blood Pressure	____	Strong Desire for Sweets/Salts	____
Moods of Depression	____	Often feel Bloated	____
Cold Hands and Feet	____	Difficulty Falling Asleep	____
Shortness of Breath	____	Allergies and/or Hayfever	____
Poor Night Vision	____	Light Sleep/Aware of Surroundings	____

NOTE: Once you have completed this health evaluation for the second time, return to the first health evaluation and compare the improvements. Make at least four extra copies of this evaluation for use once a month after you have finished the 90 Day Guide. Improvement will be gradual. By filling out the health evaluation monthly it will be easier to continue to see the progress your body is making during its healing process.

90 DAY GUIDE
DAY 1

You are embarking on one of the most exciting journeys of your life. You are taking positive steps to feeling better again. You can do it, you know you can. Enjoy the peaks you will have and know the valleys will lead to yet another higher, greater peak.

Any foods containing the following will need to be completely eliminated from your diet: Chocolate, carbonation, coffee, and alcohol. Refined sugars will need to be consumed in small quantities. We will work on eliminating these foods gradually, so you will be able to work them out of your eating habits. If it works better for you to just "cut them out," then do it. Do it the way that works best for you.

CHOCOLATE: Lower consumption to one serving daily. Number of servings today:	
CARBONATED BEVERAGES: How many cans consumed in one day? From now on, pour out 1/2 of the can so that if you drink 10 cans a day, you will now drink 10 "1/2 cans" a day. Number of "1/2 cans" consumed today:	
COFFEE: At this time, how many cups consumed in one day? From now on, pour out 1/2 of the cup so that if you drink 10 cups a day, you will now drink 10 "1/2 cups" a day. Number of "1/2 cups" consumed today:	
ALCOHOL: How many alcoholic beverages do you consume in one week? Reduce your number of alcoholic beverages to two every week. In the space write 0, 1, or 2 corresponding to the number of drinks you have had this week.	
REFINED SUGARS: Number of times refined sugars are consumed in a normal day. Beginning Today limit sugars to 2 servings per day. Number of times refined sugars consumed today:	
WATER: Drink 8 glasses of water or tea. Amount consumed today:	
EXERCISE: Walk for 5 minutes without stopping. Check the box after you walk.	
STRETCHING EXERCISE: Do exercise Plan #2 in the back of the book. Check here when finished.	
SLEEP: About 45 minutes before going to bed take a warm sage bath. Drink a cup of herbal tea. (Refer to back of book for sage bath recipe and herbal recommendations.) Read about 20 minutes while sitting in a comfortable chair. Go to bed, lie on your back and take 3-5 deep breaths. Then work the acupressure points for sleep. (Refer to the section on acupressure treatments.)	
SUPPLEMENTS: Check after taking your supplements. Breakfast: Lunch: Dinner:	
ON A SCALE OF 1-10, with 1 indicating symptom free and 10 indicating intense pain, rate how you feel today:	
Today's High Temperature:	

Briefly Describe Today's Weather:

What I Accomplished Today:

DAY 2

Today is a wonderful day! It won't be long and you will start to feel the positive effects of the work you are embarking on. Enjoy knowing you are in the healing process. If it was difficult to eliminate the foods yesterday, start again today. There is no hurry, but persistence will help you achieve your goal of feeling better.

CHOCOLATE: Maintain consumption at one serving daily. Number of servings today:	
CARBONATED BEVERAGES: Number of "1/2 cans" consumed today:	
COFFEE: Number of "1/2 cups" consumed today:	
ALCOHOL: In the space write 0, 1, or 2 corresponding to the number of drinks you have had this week.	
REFINED SUGARS: Number of times refined sugars consumed today:	
WATER: Drink 8 glasses of water or tea. Amount consumed today:	
EXERCISE: Walk for 5 minutes without stopping. Check the box after you walk.	
STRETCHING EXERCISE: Do exercise Plan #3 in the back of the book. Check the box when finished.	
SLEEP: About 45 minutes before going to bed take a warm sage bath. Drink a cup of herbal tea. (Refer to back of book for sage bath recipe and herbal recommendations.) Read about 20 minutes while sitting in a comfortable chair. Go to bed, lie on your back and take 3-5 deep breaths. Then work the acupressure points for sleep. (Refer to the section on acupressure treatments.)	
SUPPLEMENTS: Check after taking your supplements.	
Breakfast:	
Lunch:	
Dinner:	
ON A SCALE OF 1-10, with 1 indicating symptom free and 10 indicating intense pain, rate how you feel today:	
Today's High Temperature:	

Briefly Describe Today's Weather:

What I Accomplished Today:

DAY 3

I found it helpful when trying to eliminate chocolate from my diet to keep chocolate bits in the freezer. I could then keep track of how many I ate each day. (I was such a chocoholic, it took four months to kick chocolate completely!)

CHOCOLATE: Maintain consumption at one serving daily. Number of servings today:	
CARBONATED BEVERAGES: Number of "1/2 cans" consumed today:	
COFFEE: Number of "1/2 cups" consumed today:	
ALCOHOL: In the space write 0, 1, or 2 corresponding to the number of drinks you have had this week.	
REFINED SUGARS: Number of times refined sugars consumed today:	
WATER: Drink 8 glasses of water or tea. Amount consumed today:	
EXERCISE: Walk for 5 minutes without stopping. Check the box after you walk.	
STRETCHING EXERCISE: Do exercise Plan #1 in the back of the book. Check to the box when finished.	
SLEEP: About 45 minutes before going to bed take a warm sage bath. Drink a cup of herbal tea. (Refer to back of book for sage bath recipe and herbal recommendations.) Read about 20 minutes while sitting in a comfortable chair. Go to bed, lie on your back and take 3-5 deep breaths. Then work the acupressure points for sleep. (Refer to the section on acupressure treatments.)	
SUPPLEMENTS: Check after taking your supplements.	
Breakfast:	
Lunch:	
Dinner:	
ON A SCALE OF 1-10, with 1 indicating symptom free and 10 indicating intense pain, rate how you feel today:	
Today's High Temperature:	

Briefly Describe Today's Weather:

What I Accomplished Today:

DAY 4

You've made it through three days-you're doing well. Doesn't it feel good to know you are actually doing something to begin to feel better? You have finally made the choice to begin taking control of your fibromyalgia instead of it controlling you! Give yourself a pat on the back. You can do it-I know you can!

CHOCOLATE: Maintain consumption at one serving daily. Number of servings today:	
CARBONATED BEVERAGES: Number of "1/2 cans" consumed today:	
COFFEE: Number of "1/2 cups" consumed today:	
ALCOHOL: In the space write 0, 1, or 2 corresponding to the number of drinks you have had this week.	
REFINED SUGARS: Number of times refined sugars consumed today:	
WATER: Drink 8 glasses of water or tea. Amount consumed today:	
EXERCISE: Walk for 5 minutes without stopping. Check the box after you walk.	
STRETCHING EXERCISE: Do exercise Plan #1 in the back of the book. Check the box when finished.	
SLEEP: About 45 minutes before going to bed take a warm sage bath. Drink a cup of herbal tea. (Refer to back of book for sage bath recipe and herbal recommendations.) Read about 20 minutes while sitting in a comfortable chair. Go to bed, lie on your back and take 3-5 deep breaths. Then work the acupressure points for sleep. (Refer to the section on acupressure treatments.)	
SUPPLEMENTS: Check after taking your supplements.	
Breakfast:	
Lunch:	
Dinner:	
ON A SCALE OF 1-10, with 1 indicating symptom free and 10 indicating intense pain, rate how you feel today:	
Today's High Temperature:	

Briefly Describe Today's Weather:

What I Accomplished Today:

DAY 5

Each day thank your body for working with you in this healing process. This serves two purposes. First, it helps you think about getting better, not just coping. Second, it helps you start thinking healthy instead of thinking about how horrible you feel.

CHOCOLATE: Maintain consumption at one serving daily. Number of servings today:	
CARBONATED BEVERAGES: Number of "1/2 cans" consumed today:	
COFFEE: Number of "1/2 cups" consumed today:	
ALCOHOL: In the space write 0, 1, or 2 corresponding to the number of drinks you have had this week.	
REFINED SUGARS: Number of times refined sugars consumed today:	
WATER: Drink 8 glasses of water or tea. Amount consumed today:	
EXERCISE: Walk for 5 minutes without stopping. Check the box after you walk.	
STRETCHING EXERCISE: Do exercise Plan #2 in the back of the book. Check the box when finished.	
SLEEP: About 45 minutes before going to bed take a warm sage bath. Drink a cup of herbal tea. (Refer to back of book for sage bath recipe and herbal recommendations.) Read about 20 minutes while sitting in a comfortable chair. Go to bed, lie on your back and take 3-5 deep breaths. Then work the acupressure points for sleep. (Refer to the section on acupressure treatments.)	
SUPPLEMENTS: Check after taking your supplements.	
Breakfast:	
Lunch:	
Dinner:	
ON A SCALE OF 1-10, with 1 indicating symptom free and 10 indicating intense pain, rate how you feel today:	
Today's High Temperature:	

Briefly Describe Today's Weather:

What I Accomplished Today:

DAY 6

For back and shoulder pain, use some of the acupressure points in the back of the book. Many days I would do the stretching exercises more than once.

CHOCOLATE: Maintain consumption at one serving daily. Number of servings today:	
CARBONATED BEVERAGES: Number of "1/2 cans" consumed today:	
COFFEE: Number of "1/2 cups" consumed today:	
ALCOHOL: In the space write 0, 1, or 2 corresponding to the number of drinks you have had this week.	
REFINED SUGARS: Number of times refined sugars consumed today:	
WATER: Drink 8 glasses of water or tea. Amount consumed today:	
EXERCISE: Walk for 5 minutes without stopping. Check the box after you walk.	
STRETCHING EXERCISE: Do exercise Plan #3 in the back of the book. Check the box when finished.	
SLEEP: About 45 minutes before going to bed take a warm sage bath. Drink a cup of herbal tea. (Refer to back of book for sage bath recipe and herbal recommendations.) Read about 20 minutes while sitting in a comfortable chair. Go to bed, lie on your back and take 3-5 deep breaths. Then work the acupressure points for sleep. (Refer to the section on acupressure treatments.)	
SUPPLEMENTS: Check after taking your supplements.	
Breakfast:	
Lunch:	
Dinner:	
ON A SCALE OF 1-10, with 1 indicating symptom free and 10 indicating intense pain, rate how you feel today:	
Today's High Temperature:	

Briefly Describe Today's Weather:

What I Accomplished Today:

DAY 7

Take note of your posture. Be sure to stand and sit "tall." Any time you can, take deep breaths counting to seven as you inhale, filling your abdomen first, then your chest. Hold the breath for a count of five, then let it out to the count of seven.

CHOCOLATE: Maintain consumption at one serving daily. Number of servings today:	
CARBONATED BEVERAGES: Number of "1/2 cans" consumed today:	
COFFEE: Number of "1/2 cups" consumed today:	
ALCOHOL: In the space write 0, 1, or 2 corresponding to the number of drinks you have had this week.	
REFINED SUGARS: Number of times refined sugars consumed today:	
WATER: Drink 8 glasses of water or tea. Amount consumed today:	
EXERCISE: Walk for 5 minutes without stopping. Check the box after you walk.	
STRETCHING EXERCISE: Do exercise Plan #3 in the back of the book. Check the box when finished.	
SLEEP: About 45 minutes before going to bed take a warm sage bath. Drink a cup of herbal tea. (Refer to back of book for sage bath recipe and herbal recommendations.) Read about 20 minutes while sitting in a comfortable chair. Go to bed, lie on your back and take 3-5 deep breaths. Then work the acupressure points for sleep. (Refer to the section on acupressure treatments.)	
SUPPLEMENTS: Check after taking your supplements.	
Breakfast:	
Lunch:	
Dinner:	
ON A SCALE OF 1-10, with 1 indicating symptom free and 10 indicating intense pain, rate how you feel today:	
Today's High Temperature:	

Briefly Describe Today's Weather:

What I Accomplished Today:

DAY 8

You have made it through your first week! Congratulations! Keep up the good work.

CHOCOLATE: Maintain consumption at one serving daily. Number of servings today:	
CARBONATED BEVERAGES: Number of "1/2 cans" consumed today:	
COFFEE: Number of "1/2 cups" consumed today:	
ALCOHOL: In the space write 0, 1, or 2 corresponding to the number of drinks you have had this week.	
REFINED SUGARS: Number of times refined sugars consumed today:	
WATER: Drink 8 glasses of water or tea. Amount consumed today:	
EXERCISE: Walk for 5 minutes without stopping. Check the box after you walk.	
STRETCHING EXERCISE: Do exercise Plan #1 in the back of the book. Check the box when finished.	
SLEEP: About 45 minutes before going to bed take a warm sage bath. Drink a cup of herbal tea. (Refer to back of book for sage bath recipe and herbal recommendations.) Read about 20 minutes while sitting in a comfortable chair. Go to bed, lie on your back and take 3-5 deep breaths. Then work the acupressure points for sleep. (Refer to the section on acupressure treatments.)	
SUPPLEMENTS: Check after taking your supplements.	
Breakfast:	
Lunch:	
Dinner:	
ON A SCALE OF 1-10, with 1 indicating symptom free and 10 indicating intense pain, rate how you feel today:	
Today's High Temperature:	

Briefly Describe Today's Weather:

What I Accomplished Today:

DAY 9

Today pick one hour and try to judge nothing during that hour. By being non-judgmental, your mind has a chance to rest and restore itself. This is very important to help the body heal.

CHOCOLATE: Maintain consumption at one serving daily. Number of servings today:	
CARBONATED BEVERAGES: Number of "1/2 cans" consumed today:	
COFFEE: Number of "1/2 cups" consumed today:	
ALCOHOL: In the space write 0, 1, or 2 corresponding to the number of drinks you have had this week.	
REFINED SUGARS: Number of times refined sugars consumed today:	
WATER: Drink 8 glasses of water or tea. Amount consumed today:	
EXERCISE: Walk for 5 minutes without stopping. Check the box after you walk.	
STRETCHING EXERCISE: Do exercise Plan #2 in the back of the book. Check the box when finished.	
SLEEP: About 45 minutes before going to bed take a warm sage bath. Drink a cup of herbal tea. (Refer to back of book for sage bath recipe and herbal recommendations.) Read about 20 minutes while sitting in a comfortable chair. Go to bed, lie on your back and take 3-5 deep breaths. Then work the acupressure points for sleep. (Refer to the section on acupressure treatments.)	
SUPPLEMENTS: Check after taking your supplements.	
Breakfast:	
Lunch:	
Dinner:	
ON A SCALE OF 1-10, with 1 indicating symptom free and 10 indicating intense pain, rate how you feel today:	
Today's High Temperature:	

Briefly Describe Today's Weather:

What I Accomplished Today:

DAY 10

Today, as you begin your day, stand up tall, and stretch your arms out to the side, take a deep breath, and thank your body for the healing process taking place within it. Then stretch your arms above your head as far as possible and take another deep breath.

CHOCOLATE: Maintain consumption at one serving daily. Number of servings today:	
CARBONATED BEVERAGES: Number of "1/2 cans" consumed today:	
COFFEE: Number of "1/2 cups" consumed today:	
ALCOHOL: In the space write 0, 1, or 2 corresponding to the number of drinks you have had this week.	
REFINED SUGARS: Number of times refined sugars consumed today:	
WATER: Drink 8 glasses of water or tea. Amount consumed today:	
EXERCISE: Walk for 5 minutes without stopping. Check the box after you walk.	
STRETCHING EXERCISE: Do exercise Plan #3 in the back of the book. Check the box when finished.	
SLEEP: About 45 minutes before going to bed take a warm sage bath. Drink a cup of herbal tea. (Refer to back of book for sage bath recipe and herbal recommendations.) Read about 20 minutes while sitting in a comfortable chair. Go to bed, lie on your back and take 3-5 deep breaths. Then work the acupressure points for sleep. (Refer to the section on acupressure treatments.)	
SUPPLEMENTS: Check after taking your supplements.	
Breakfast:	
Lunch:	
Dinner:	
ON A SCALE OF 1-10, with 1 indicating symptom free and 10 indicating intense pain, rate how you feel today.	
Today's High Temperature:	

Briefly Describe Today's Weather:

What I Accomplished Today:

DAY 11

It is so important to eat plenty of fresh fruits and vegetables. It is believed our bodies do not metabolize foods in the same manner as a "healthy" body. With that in mind, we need the additional nutritional value from fresh foods that we may not get from processed or canned foods.

CHOCOLATE: Maintain consumption at one serving daily. Number of servings today:	
CARBONATED BEVERAGES: Number of "1/2 cans" consumed today:	
COFFEE: Number of "1/2 cups" consumed today:	
ALCOHOL: In the space write 0, 1, or 2 corresponding to the number of drinks you have had this week.	
REFINED SUGARS: Number of times refined sugars consumed today:	
WATER: Drink 8 glasses of water or tea. Amount consumed today:	
EXERCISE: Walk for 5 minutes without stopping. Check the box after you walk.	
STRETCHING EXERCISE: Do exercise Plan #2 in the back of the book. Check the box when finished.	
SLEEP: About 45 minutes before going to bed take a warm sage bath. Drink a cup of herbal tea. (Refer to back of book for sage bath recipe and herbal recommendations.) Read about 20 minutes while sitting in a comfortable chair. Go to bed, lie on your back and take 3-5 deep breaths. Then work the acupressure points for sleep. (Refer to the section on acupressure treatments.)	
SUPPLEMENTS: Check after taking your supplements.	
Breakfast:	
Lunch:	
Dinner:	
ON A SCALE OF 1-10, with 1 indicating symptom free and 10 indicating intense pain, rate how you feel today:	
Today's High Temperature:	

Briefly Describe Today's Weather:

What I Accomplished Today:

DAY 12

If you slip on a day, don't beat yourself up. Know that tomorrow's another day and you can begin again fresh.

CHOCOLATE: Maintain consumption at one serving daily. Number of servings today:	
CARBONATED BEVERAGES: Number of "1/2 cans" consumed today:	
COFFEE: Number of "1/2 cups" consumed today:	
ALCOHOL: In the space write 0, 1, or 2 corresponding to the number of drinks you have had this week.	
REFINED SUGARS: Number of times refined sugars consumed today:	
WATER: Drink 8 glasses of water or tea. Amount consumed today:	
EXERCISE: Walk for 5 minutes without stopping. Check the box after you walk.	
STRETCHING EXERCISE: Do exercise Plan #2 in the back of the book. Check the box when finished.	
SLEEP: About 45 minutes before going to bed take a warm sage bath. Drink a cup of herbal tea. (Refer to back of book for sage bath recipe and herbal recommendations.) Read about 20 minutes while sitting in a comfortable chair. Go to bed, lie on your back and take 3-5 deep breaths. Then work the acupressure points for sleep. (Refer to the section on acupressure treatments.)	
SUPPLEMENTS: Check after taking your supplements.	
Breakfast:	
Lunch:	
Dinner:	
ON A SCALE OF 1-10, with 1 indicating symptom free and 10 indicating intense pain, rate how you feel today:	
Today's High Temperature:	

Briefly Describe Today's Weather:

What I Accomplished Today:

DAY 13

During the day today, try to think positively about anything you may normally think of as being a negative in your life. I always wondered why I had to get FMS, however, after 35 years I can finally see that this is what I needed to go through to be able to help you feel better.

CHOCOLATE: Maintain consumption at one serving daily. Number of servings today:	
CARBONATED BEVERAGES: Number of "1/2 cans" consumed today:	
COFFEE: Number of "1/2 cups" consumed today:	
ALCOHOL: In the space write 0, 1, or 2 corresponding to the number of drinks you have had this week.	
REFINED SUGARS: Number of times refined sugars consumed today:	
WATER: Drink 8 glasses of water or tea. Amount consumed today:	
EXERCISE: Walk for 5 minutes without stopping. Check the box after you walk.	
STRETCHING EXERCISE: Do exercise Plan #3 in the back of the book. Check the box when finished.	
SLEEP: About 45 minutes before going to bed take a warm sage bath. Drink a cup of herbal tea. (Refer to back of book for sage bath recipe and herbal recommendations.) Read about 20 minutes while sitting in a comfortable chair. Go to bed, lie on your back and take 3-5 deep breaths. Then work the acupressure points for sleep. (Refer to the section on acupressure treatments.)	
SUPPLEMENTS: Check after taking your supplements.	
Breakfast:	
Lunch:	
Dinner:	
ON A SCALE OF 1-10, with 1 indicating symptom free and 10 indicating intense pain, rate how you feel today:	
Today's High Temperature:	

Briefly Describe Today's Weather:

What I Accomplished Today:

DAY 14

I have found over the years that once I started embracing life, it started embracing me. What a wonderful feeling!

CHOCOLATE: Maintain consumption at one serving daily. Number of servings today:	
CARBONATED BEVERAGES: Number of "1/2 cans" consumed today:	
COFFEE: Number of "1/2 cups" consumed today:	
ALCOHOL: In the space write 0, 1, or 2 corresponding to the number of drinks you have had this week.	
REFINED SUGARS: Number of times refined sugars consumed today:	
WATER: Drink 8 glasses of water or tea. Amount consumed today:	
EXERCISE: Walk for 5 minutes without stopping. Check the box after you walk.	
STRETCHING EXERCISE: Do exercise Plan #1 in the back of the book. Check the box when finished.	
SLEEP: About 45 minutes before going to bed take a warm sage bath. Drink a cup of herbal tea. (Refer to back of book for sage bath recipe and herbal recommendations.) Read about 20 minutes while sitting in a comfortable chair. Go to bed, lie on your back and take 3-5 deep breaths. Then work the acupressure points for sleep. (Refer to the section on acupressure treatments.)	
SUPPLEMENTS: Check after taking your supplements.	
Breakfast:	
Lunch:	
Dinner:	
ON A SCALE OF 1-10, with 1 indicating symptom free and 10 indicating intense pain, rate how you feel today:	
Today's High Temperature:	

Briefly Describe Today's Weather:

What I Accomplished Today:

DAY 15

If FMS is caused from a buildup of toxins, it would be to our benefit to stay away from as many toxic chemicals as possible. Instead of using insecticides to keep ants from coming into your house, try making a strong tea from garlic and spray that around the base of your house.

CHOCOLATE: Maintain consumption at one serving daily. Number of servings today:	
CARBONATED BEVERAGES: Number of "1/2 cans" consumed today:	
COFFEE: Number of "1/2 cups" consumed today:	
ALCOHOL: In the space write 0, 1, or 2 corresponding to the number of drinks you have had this week.	
REFINED SUGARS: Number of times refined sugars consumed today:	
WATER: Drink 8 glasses of water or tea. Amount consumed today:	
EXERCISE: Walk for 5 minutes without stopping. Check the box after you walk.	
STRETCHING EXERCISE: Do exercise Plan #2 in the back of the book. Check the box when finished.	
SLEEP: About 45 minutes before going to bed take a warm sage bath. Drink a cup of herbal tea. (Refer to back of book for sage bath recipe and herbal recommendations.) Read about 20 minutes while sitting in a comfortable chair. Go to bed, lie on your back and take 3-5 deep breaths. Then work the acupressure points for sleep. (Refer to the section on acupressure treatments.)	
SUPPLEMENTS: Check after taking your supplements.	
Breakfast:	
Lunch:	
Dinner:	
ON A SCALE OF 1-10, with 1 indicating symptom free and 10 indicating intense pain, rate how you feel today:	
Today's High Temperature:	

Briefly Describe Today's Weather:

What I Accomplished Today:

DAY 16

Can you believe you have already been working on becoming healthy for more than two weeks? Concentrate on how good it will feel to do the things you like to do again, and use those thoughts to give yourself strength.

CHOCOLATE: Maintain consumption at one serving daily. Number of servings today:	
CARBONATED BEVERAGES: Number of "1/2 cans" consumed today:	
COFFEE: Number of "1/2 cups" consumed today:	
ALCOHOL: In the space write 0, 1, or 2 corresponding to the number of drinks you have had this week.	
REFINED SUGARS: Number of times refined sugars consumed today:	
WATER: Drink 8 glasses of water or tea. Amount consumed today:	
EXERCISE: Walk for 5 minutes without stopping. Check the box after you walk.	
STRETCHING EXERCISE: Do exercise Plan #3 in the back of the book. Check the box when finished.	
SLEEP: About 45 minutes before going to bed take a warm sage bath. Drink a cup of herbal tea. (Refer to back of book for sage bath recipe and herbal recommendations.) Read about 20 minutes while sitting in a comfortable chair. Go to bed, lie on your back and take 3-5 deep breaths. Then work the acupressure points for sleep. (Refer to the section on acupressure treatments.)	
SUPPLEMENTS: Check after taking your supplements.	
Breakfast:	
Lunch:	
Dinner:	
ON A SCALE OF 1-10, with 1 indicating symptom free and 10 indicating intense pain, rate how you feel today:	
Today's High Temperature:	

Briefly Describe Today's Weather:

What I Accomplished Today:

DAY 17

If you notice a sore throat coming on, gargle with saltwater. A good solution is made with one teaspoon salt in 1/4 cup of warm water. Gargle four times per day.

CHOCOLATE: Maintain consumption at one serving daily. Number of servings today:	
CARBONATED BEVERAGES: Number of "1/2 cans" consumed today:	
COFFEE: Number of "1/2 cups" consumed today:	
ALCOHOL: In the space write 0, 1, or 2 corresponding to the number of drinks you have had this week.	
REFINED SUGARS: Number of times refined sugars consumed today:	
WATER: Drink 8 glasses of water or tea. Amount consumed today:	
EXERCISE: Walk for 5 minutes without stopping. Check the box after you walk.	
STRETCHING EXERCISE: Do exercise Plan #1 in the back of the book. Check the box when finished.	
SLEEP: About 45 minutes before going to bed take a warm sage bath. Drink a cup of herbal tea. (Refer to back of book for sage bath recipe and herbal recommendations.) Read about 20 minutes while sitting in a comfortable chair. Go to bed, lie on your back and take 3-5 deep breaths. Then work the acupressure points for sleep. (Refer to the section on acupressure treatments.)	
SUPPLEMENTS: Check after taking your supplements.	
Breakfast:	
Lunch:	
Dinner:	
ON A SCALE OF 1-10, with 1 indicating symptom free and 10 indicating intense pain, rate how you feel today:	
Today's High Temperature:	

Briefly Describe Today's Weather:

What I Accomplished Today:

DAY 18

When a virus seems to be coming on, many times it can be headed off by drinking echinacea tea. Echinacea can be obtained from most health food stores.

CHOCOLATE: Maintain consumption at one serving daily. Number of servings today:	
CARBONATED BEVERAGES: Number of "1/2 cans" consumed today:	
COFFEE: Number of "1/2 cups" consumed today:	
ALCOHOL: In the space write 0, 1, or 2 corresponding to the number of drinks you have had this week.	
REFINED SUGARS: Number of times refined sugars consumed today:	
WATER: Drink 8 glasses of water or tea. Amount consumed today:	
EXERCISE: Walk for 5 minutes without stopping. Check the box after you walk.	
STRETCHING EXERCISE: Do exercise Plan #2 in the back of the book. Check the box when finished.	
SLEEP: About 45 minutes before going to bed take a warm sage bath. Drink a cup of herbal tea. (Refer to back of book for sage bath recipe and herbal recommendations.) Read about 20 minutes while sitting in a comfortable chair. Go to bed, lie on your back and take 3-5 deep breaths. Then work the acupressure points for sleep. (Refer to the section on acupressure treatments.)	
SUPPLEMENTS: Check after taking your supplements.	
Breakfast:	
Lunch:	
Dinner:	
ON A SCALE OF 1-10, with 1 indicating symptom free and 10 indicating intense pain, rate how you feel today:	
Today's High Temperature:	

Briefly Describe Today's Weather:

What I Accomplished Today:

DAY 19

White flour breaks down in the body to a form similar to that of white sugar. Try to limit the amount of white breads you eat to one per meal.

CHOCOLATE: Maintain consumption at one serving daily. Number of servings today:	
CARBONATED BEVERAGES: Number of "1/2 cans" consumed today:	
COFFEE: Number of "1/2 cups" consumed today:	
ALCOHOL: In the space write 0, 1, or 2 corresponding to the number of drinks you have had this week.	
REFINED SUGARS: Number of times refined sugars consumed today:	
WATER: Drink 8 glasses of water or tea. Amount consumed today:	
EXERCISE: Walk for 5 minutes without stopping. Check the box after you walk.	
STRETCHING EXERCISE: Do exercise Plan #3 in the back of the book. Check the box when finished.	
SLEEP: About 45 minutes before going to bed take a warm sage bath. Drink a cup of herbal tea. (Refer to back of book for sage bath recipe and herbal recommendations.) Read about 20 minutes while sitting in a comfortable chair. Go to bed, lie on your back and take 3-5 deep breaths. Then work the acupressure points for sleep. (Refer to the section on acupressure treatments.)	
SUPPLEMENTS: Check after taking your supplements.	
Breakfast:	
Lunch:	
Dinner:	
ON A SCALE OF 1-10, with 1 indicating symptom free and 10 indicating intense pain, rate how you feel today:	
Today's High Temperature:	

Briefly Describe Today's Weather:

What I Accomplished Today:

DAY 20

Today, after you record your accomplishments, write one goal you would like to achieve when you are feeling better. Hold that goal in your mind, and know you will eventually reach it.

CHOCOLATE: Maintain consumption at one serving daily. Number of servings today:	
CARBONATED BEVERAGES: Number of "1/2 cans" consumed today:	
COFFEE: Number of "1/2 cups" consumed today:	
ALCOHOL: In the space write 0, 1, or 2 corresponding to the number of drinks you have had this week.	
REFINED SUGARS: Number of times refined sugars consumed today:	
WATER: Drink 8 glasses of water or tea. Amount consumed today:	
EXERCISE: Walk for 5 minutes without stopping. Check the box after you walk.	
STRETCHING EXERCISE: Do exercise Plan #1 in the back of the book. Check the box when finished.	
SLEEP: About 45 minutes before going to bed take a warm sage bath. Drink a cup of herbal tea. (Refer to back of book for sage bath recipe and herbal recommendations.) Read about 20 minutes while sitting in a comfortable chair. Go to bed, lie on your back and take 3-5 deep breaths. Then work the acupressure points for sleep. (Refer to the section on acupressure treatments.)	
SUPPLEMENTS: Check after taking your supplements.	
Breakfast:	
Lunch:	
Dinner:	
ON A SCALE OF 1-10, with 1 indicating symptom free and 10 indicating intense pain, rate how you feel today:	
Today's High Temperature:	

Briefly Describe Today's Weather:

What I Accomplished Today:

DAY 21

It is not uncommon after having a few good days to fall back into a form of relapse, which many times seems as bad as before you began the program. Continue on the program and you will start to feel better.

CHOCOLATE: Maintain consumption at one serving daily. Number of servings today:	
CARBONATED BEVERAGES: Number of "1/2 cans" consumed today:	
COFFEE: Number of "1/2 cups" consumed today:	
ALCOHOL: In the space write 0, 1, or 2 corresponding to the number of drinks you have had this week.	
REFINED SUGARS: Number of times refined sugars consumed today:	
WATER: Drink 8 glasses of water or tea. Amount consumed today:	
EXERCISE: Walk for 5 minutes without stopping. Check the box after you walk.	
STRETCHING EXERCISE: Do exercise Plan #2 in the back of the book. Check the box when finished.	
SLEEP: About 45 minutes before going to bed take a warm sage bath. Drink a cup of herbal tea. (Refer to back of book for sage bath recipe and herbal recommendations.) Read about 20 minutes while sitting in a comfortable chair. Go to bed, lie on your back and take 3-5 deep breaths. Then work the acupressure points for sleep. (Refer to the section on acupressure treatments.)	
SUPPLEMENTS: Check after taking your supplements.	
Breakfast:	
Lunch:	
Dinner:	
ON A SCALE OF 1-10, with 1 indicating symptom free and 10 indicating intense pain, rate how you feel today:	
Today's High Temperature:	

Briefly Describe Today's Weather:

What I Accomplished Today:

DAY 22

Instead of looking for that front parking space, begin parking farther out in the parking lot and walking the extra distance.

CHOCOLATE: Maintain consumption at one serving daily. Number of servings today:	
CARBONATED BEVERAGES: Number of "1/2 cans" consumed today:	
COFFEE: Number of "1/2 cups" consumed today:	
ALCOHOL: In the space write 0, 1, or 2 corresponding to the number of drinks you have had this week.	
REFINED SUGARS: Number of times refined sugars consumed today:	
WATER: Drink 8 glasses of water or tea. Amount consumed today:	
EXERCISE: Walk for 5 minutes without stopping. Check the box after you walk.	
STRETCHING EXERCISE: Do exercise Plan #3 in the back of the book. Check the box when finished.	
SLEEP: About 45 minutes before going to bed take a warm sage bath. Drink a cup of herbal tea. (Refer to back of book for sage bath recipe and herbal recommendations.) Read about 20 minutes while sitting in a comfortable chair. Go to bed, lie on your back and take 3-5 deep breaths. Then work the acupressure points for sleep. (Refer to the section on acupressure treatments.)	
SUPPLEMENTS: Check after taking your supplements.	
Breakfast:	
Lunch:	
Dinner:	
ON A SCALE OF 1-10, with 1 indicating symptom free and 10 indicating intense pain, rate how you feel today:	
Today's High Temperature:	

Briefly Describe Today's Weather:

What I Accomplished Today:

DAY 23

Believe within your heart, with all your being, that you will be healthy again. Any time there is a doubt in your mind, simply remind yourself you are becoming healthy again.

CHOCOLATE: Maintain consumption at one serving daily. Number of servings today:	
CARBONATED BEVERAGES: Number of "1/2 cans" consumed today:	
COFFEE: Number of "1/2 cups" consumed today:	
ALCOHOL: In the space write 0, 1, or 2 corresponding to the number of drinks you have had this week.	
REFINED SUGARS: Number of times refined sugars consumed today:	
WATER: Drink 8 glasses of water or tea. Amount consumed today:	
EXERCISE: Walk for 5 minutes without stopping. Check the box after you walk.	
STRETCHING EXERCISE: Do exercise Plan #1 in the back of the book. Check the box when finished.	
SLEEP: About 45 minutes before going to bed take a warm sage bath. Drink a cup of herbal tea. (Refer to back of book for sage bath recipe and herbal recommendations.) Read about 20 minutes while sitting in a comfortable chair. Go to bed, lie on your back and take 3-5 deep breaths. Then work the acupressure points for sleep. (Refer to the section on acupressure treatments.)	
SUPPLEMENTS: Check after taking your supplements.	
Breakfast:	
Lunch:	
Dinner:	
ON A SCALE OF 1-10, with 1 indicating symptom free and 10 indicating intense pain, rate how you feel today:	
Today's High Temperature:	

Briefly Describe Today's Weather:

What I Accomplished Today:

DAY 24

Walking is actually good for pain control. When walking, many of the large muscles in the back, legs and arms are used. This movement can help reduce pain throughout the body.

CHOCOLATE: Maintain consumption at one serving daily. Number of servings today:	
CARBONATED BEVERAGES: Number of "1/2 cans" consumed today:	
COFFEE: Number of "1/2 cups" consumed today:	
ALCOHOL: In the space write 0, 1, or 2 corresponding to the number of drinks you have had this week.	
REFINED SUGARS: Number of times refined sugars consumed today:	
WATER: Drink 8 glasses of water or tea. Amount consumed today:	
EXERCISE: Walk for 5 minutes without stopping. Check the box after you walk.	
STRETCHING EXERCISE: Do exercise Plan #2 in the back of the book. Check the box when finished.	
SLEEP: About 45 minutes before going to bed take a warm sage bath. Drink a cup of herbal tea. (Refer to back of book for sage bath recipe and herbal recommendations.) Read about 20 minutes while sitting in a comfortable chair. Go to bed, lie on your back and take 3-5 deep breaths. Then work the acupressure points for sleep. (Refer to the section on acupressure treatments.)	
SUPPLEMENTS: Check after taking your supplements.	
Breakfast:	
Lunch:	
Dinner:	
ON A SCALE OF 1-10, with 1 indicating symptom free and 10 indicating intense pain, rate how you feel today:	
Today's High Temperature:	

Briefly Describe Today's Weather:

What I Accomplished Today:

DAY 25

Garlic is a natural antibiotic, although caution should be used when taking it since it can also lower blood pressure.

CHOCOLATE: Maintain consumption at one serving daily. Number of servings today:	
CARBONATED BEVERAGES: Number of "1/2 cans" consumed today:	
COFFEE: Number of "1/2 cups" consumed today:	
ALCOHOL: In the space write 0, 1, or 2 corresponding to the number of drinks you have had this week.	
REFINED SUGARS: Number of times refined sugars consumed today:	
WATER: Drink 8 glasses of water or tea. Amount consumed today:	
EXERCISE: Walk for 5 minutes without stopping. Check the box after you walk.	
STRETCHING EXERCISE: Do exercise Plan #3 in the back of the book. Check the box when finished.	
SLEEP: About 45 minutes before going to bed take a warm sage bath. Drink a cup of herbal tea. (Refer to back of book for sage bath recipe and herbal recommendations.) Read about 20 minutes while sitting in a comfortable chair. Go to bed, lie on your back and take 3-5 deep breaths. Then work the acupressure points for sleep. (Refer to the section on acupressure treatments.)	
SUPPLEMENTS: Check after taking your supplements.	
Breakfast:	
Lunch:	
Dinner:	
ON A SCALE OF 1-10, with 1 indicating symptom free and 10 indicating intense pain, rate how you feel today:	
Today's High Temperature:	

Briefly Describe Today's Weather:

What I Accomplished Today:

DAY 26

Echinacea is also a natural antibiotic and immune booster. This perennial herb is better known as "coneflower."

CHOCOLATE: Maintain consumption at one serving daily. Number of servings today:	
CARBONATED BEVERAGES: Number of "1/2 cans" consumed today:	
COFFEE: Number of "1/2 cups" consumed today:	
ALCOHOL: In the space write 0, 1, or 2 corresponding to the number of drinks you have had this week.	
REFINED SUGARS: Number of times refined sugars consumed today:	
WATER: Drink 8 glasses of water or tea. Amount consumed today:	
EXERCISE: Walk for 5 minutes without stopping. Check the box after you walk.	
STRETCHING EXERCISE: Do exercise Plan #1 in the back of the book. Check the box when finished.	
SLEEP: About 45 minutes before going to bed take a warm sage bath. Drink a cup of herbal tea. (Refer to back of book for sage bath recipe and herbal recommendations.) Read about 20 minutes while sitting in a comfortable chair. Go to bed, lie on your back and take 3-5 deep breaths. Then work the acupressure points for sleep. (Refer to the section on acupressure treatments.)	
SUPPLEMENTS: Check after taking your supplements.	
Breakfast:	
Lunch:	
Dinner:	
ON A SCALE OF 1-10, with 1 indicating symptom free and 10 indicating intense pain, rate how you feel today:	
Today's High Temperature:	

Briefly Describe Today's Weather:

What I Accomplished Today:

DAY 27

Approximately 20 percent of Americans are believed to have FMS, although only about 7 percent have been diagnosed.

CHOCOLATE: Maintain consumption at one serving daily. Number of servings today:	
CARBONATED BEVERAGES: Number of "1/2 cans" consumed today:	
COFFEE: Number of "1/2 cups" consumed today:	
ALCOHOL: In the space write 0, 1, or 2 corresponding to the number of drinks you have had this week.	
REFINED SUGARS: Number of times refined sugars consumed today:	
WATER: Drink 8 glasses of water or tea. Amount consumed today:	
EXERCISE: Walk for 5 minutes without stopping. Check the box after you walk.	
STRETCHING EXERCISE: Do exercise Plan #2 in the back of the book. Check the box when finished.	
SLEEP: About 45 minutes before going to bed take a warm sage bath. Drink a cup of herbal tea. (Refer to back of book for sage bath recipe and herbal recommendations.) Read about 20 minutes while sitting in a comfortable chair. Go to bed, lie on your back and take 3-5 deep breaths. Then work the acupressure points for sleep. (Refer to the section on acupressure treatments.)	
SUPPLEMENTS: Check after taking your supplements.	
Breakfast:	
Lunch:	
Dinner:	
ON A SCALE OF 1-10, with 1 indicating symptom free and 10 indicating intense pain, rate how you feel today:	
Today's High Temperature:	

Briefly Describe Today's Weather:

What I Accomplished Today:

DAY 28

Most whole wheat breads are more nutritious than white breads because they are processed less. Many other flours can be used for baking instead of white flours. Some of these include brown rice flour, amaranth flour, and oat flour. The texture in baked goods will be a little different, but these flours are very healthy and do not break down in the same manner in our systems as white flours do.

CHOCOLATE: Maintain consumption at one serving daily. Number of servings today:	
CARBONATED BEVERAGES: Number of "1/2 cans" consumed today:	
COFFEE: Number of "1/2 cups" consumed today:	
ALCOHOL: In the space write 0, 1, or 2 corresponding to the number of drinks you have had this week.	
REFINED SUGARS: Number of times refined sugars consumed today:	
WATER: Drink 8 glasses of water or tea. Amount consumed today:	
EXERCISE: Walk for 5 minutes without stopping. Check the box after you walk.	
STRETCHING EXERCISE: Do exercise Plan #3 in the back of the book. Check the box when finished.	
SLEEP: About 45 minutes before going to bed take a warm sage bath. Drink a cup of herbal tea. (Refer to back of book for sage bath recipe and herbal recommendations.) Read about 20 minutes while sitting in a comfortable chair. Go to bed, lie on your back and take 3-5 deep breaths. Then work the acupressure points for sleep. (Refer to the section on acupressure treatments.)	
SUPPLEMENTS: Check after taking your supplements.	
Breakfast:	
Lunch:	
Dinner:	
ON A SCALE OF 1-10, with 1 indicating symptom free and 10 indicating intense pain, rate how you feel today:	
Today's High Temperature:	

Briefly Describe Today's Weather:

What I Accomplished Today:

DAY 29

You've worked very hard. Do something nice for yourself today.

CHOCOLATE: Maintain consumption at one serving daily. Number of servings today:	
CARBONATED BEVERAGES: Number of "1/2 cans" consumed today:	
COFFEE: Number of "1/2 cups" consumed today:	
ALCOHOL: In the space write 0, 1, or 2 corresponding to the number of drinks you have had this week.	
REFINED SUGARS: Number of times refined sugars consumed today:	
WATER: Drink 8 glasses of water or tea. Amount consumed today:	
EXERCISE: Walk for 5 minutes without stopping. Check the box after you walk.	
STRETCHING EXERCISE: Do exercise Plan #1 in the back of the book. Check the box when finished.	
SLEEP: About 45 minutes before going to bed take a warm sage bath. Drink a cup of herbal tea. (Refer to back of book for sage bath recipe and herbal recommendations.) Read about 20 minutes while sitting in a comfortable chair. Go to bed, lie on your back and take 3-5 deep breaths. Then work the acupressure points for sleep. (Refer to the section on acupressure treatments.)	
SUPPLEMENTS: Check after taking your supplements.	
Breakfast:	
Lunch:	
Dinner:	
ON A SCALE OF 1-10, with 1 indicating symptom free and 10 indicating intense pain, rate how you feel today:	
Today's High Temperature:	

Briefly Describe Today's Weather:

What I Accomplished Today:

DAY 30

You've reached a milestone in your journey. It takes approximately 30 days to change a habit. You are well on your way to creating a healthier, happier life!

CHOCOLATE: Maintain consumption at one serving daily. Number of servings today:	
CARBONATED BEVERAGES: Number of "1/2 cans" consumed today:	
COFFEE: Number of "1/2 cups" consumed today:	
ALCOHOL: In the space write 0, 1, or 2 corresponding to the number of drinks you have had this week.	
REFINED SUGARS: Number of times refined sugars consumed today:	
WATER: Drink 8 glasses of water or tea. Amount consumed today:	
EXERCISE: Walk for 5 minutes without stopping. Check the box after you walk.	
STRETCHING EXERCISE: Do exercise Plan #2 in the back of the book. Check the box when finished.	
SLEEP: About 45 minutes before going to bed take a warm sage bath. Drink a cup of herbal tea. (Refer to back of book for sage bath recipe and herbal recommendations.) Read about 20 minutes while sitting in a comfortable chair. Go to bed, lie on your back and take 3-5 deep breaths. Then work the acupressure points for sleep. (Refer to the section on acupressure treatments.)	
SUPPLEMENTS: Check after taking your supplements.	
Breakfast:	
Lunch:	
Dinner:	
ON A SCALE OF 1-10, with 1 indicating symptom free and 10 indicating intense pain, rate how you feel today:	
Today's High Temperature:	

Briefly Describe Today's Weather:

What I Accomplished Today:

HEALTH EVALUATION FORM

Indicate in the column next to the symptoms which of the following conditions apply to you in terms of frequency and/or intensity of symptoms using the numbers of 1-10: With 1 indicating the least and 10 indicating the greatest intensity or frequency.

Low Energy ____	Often Feel Tired ____	Headaches ____
Dry/Itchy Skin ____	Dry or Itchy Scalp ____	Rashes or Eczema ____
Achy Joints ____	Muscle Cramps ____	Muscle Twitches ____
Bruising ____	Menstrual Cramps ____	Moody/PMS ____
Poor Concentration____	Water Retention ____	Bowel Gas ____
Numbing/Tingling____	Skin Burning ____	Dry Eyes ____
Weak Fingernails ____	Dry/Brittle Hair ____	Weak Muscles ____
Joint Pain ____	Foot Pain ____	TMJ Pain ____

Indigestion/Acid Reflux ____	Constipation and/or Diarrhea ____
Frequently Take Pain Killers ____	Difficulty Handling Stress ____
High/Low Blood Pressure ____	Strong Desire for Sweets/Salts ____
Moods of Depression ____	Often feel Bloated ____
Cold Hands and Feet ____	Difficulty Falling Asleep ____
Shortness of Breath ____	Allergies and/or Hayfever ____
Poor Night Vision ____	Light Sleep/Aware of Surroundings ____

NOTE: Once you have completed this health evaluation, return to the first health evaluation and compare the improvements. Make at least four extra copies of this evaluation for use once a month after you have finished the 90 Day Guide. Improvement will be gradual. By filling out the health evaluation monthly it will be easier to continue to see the progress your body is making during its healing process.

My Gift to You

I tried to climb the mountaintop of prosperity,
But each time came tumbling down,
thinking God had forgotten me.
And each time I came tumbling down
the pain would get stronger
Until at last, I gave in, and knew I needed longer.
To learn the things nature held in her hand,
asking me to try each, and every
one until I learned why.
Each time I came tumbling down that mountaintop was a lesson,
I was to take out to the world, to help each and every person
Who, like me, was having pain.
And give the hope into their hearts
That they too, could feed good again.
So, my friend, my gift to you is to know someone cares
To see you once again climbing the hill to health.
And knowing all the while you'll be in my prayers.

Mary Moeller

DAY 31

We will begin working on increasing exercise during this next 30 days to help create deeper sleep and diminished pain.

CHOCOLATE: Starting today you will reduce your chocolate consumption to one serving every other day. Reduce serving size to half that of Day 30. Note amount eaten today:	
CARBONATED BEVERAGES: Today cut your number of cans per day in half, so that if you were drinking 10 "1/2 cans," you will now be drinking 5 "1/2 cans." Number of "1/2 cans" consumed today:	
COFFEE: Today cut your number of cups per day in half, so that if you were drinking 10 "1/2 cups," you will now be drinking 5 "1/2 cups." Number of "1/2 cups" consumed today:	
ALCOHOL: Allow yourself alcoholic beverages two times every two weeks. In the space write 0, 1, or 2 corresponding to the number of drinks you have had.	
REFINED SUGARS: Limit sugars to 1 serving and white bread to 2 servings. Enter the amount consumed today:	
WATER: Drink 8 glasses of water. Amount consumed today:	
EXERCISE: Walk 20 minutes without stopping. Check here when finished.	
STRETCHING EXERCISE: Do exercise Plan #2 in the back of the book. Check the box when finished.	
SLEEP: About 45 minutes before going to bed take a warm sage bath. Drink a cup of herbal tea. (Refer to back of book for sage bath recipe and herbal recommendations.) Read for about 20 minutes while sitting in a comfortable chair. Go to bed, lie on your back and take 3-5 deep breaths. Then work the acupressure points for sleep.	
SUPPLEMENTS: Check after taking your supplements.	
Breakfast:	
Lunch:	
Dinner:	
ON A SCALE OF 1-10, with 1 indicating symptom free and 10 indicating intense pain, rate how you feel today:	
Today's High Temperature:	

Briefly Describe Today's Weather:

What I Accomplished Today:

DAY 32

Decaffeinated coffee is just as detrimental to our systems as regular coffee.

CHOCOLATE: Maintain consumption at one serving every other day. And please remember, the serving should be half the size that it was in the previous 30 day period. Indicate, with a 0 or 1, the amount eaten today:	
CARBONATED BEVERAGES: Number of "1/2 cans" consumed today:	
COFFEE: Number of "1/2 cups" consumed today:	
ALCOHOL: Allow yourself alcoholic beverages two times every two weeks. In the space write 0, 1 or 2 corresponding to the number consumed in this two week period.	
REFINED SUGARS: Limit sugars to 1 serving and white bread to 2 servings. Enter amount consumed today:	
WATER: Drink 8 glasses of water or tea. Amount consumed today:	
EXERCISE: Walk 20 minutes without stopping. Check here when finished.	
STRETCHING EXERCISE: Do exercise Plan #2 in the back of the book. Check the box when finished.	
SLEEP: About 45 minutes before going to bed take a warm sage bath. Drink a cup of herbal tea. Read for about 20 minutes while sitting in a comfortable chair. Go to bed, lie on your back and take 3-5 deep breaths. Then work the acupressure points for sleep.	
SUPPLEMENTS: Check after taking your supplements.	
Breakfast:	
Lunch:	
Dinner:	
ON A SCALE OF 1-10, with 1 indicating symptom free and 10 indicating intense pain, rate how you feel today:	
Today's High Temperature:	

Briefly Describe Today's Weather:

What I Accomplished Today:

DAY 33

A great replacement for carbonated beverages is a glass of ice cold water with lemon in it.

CHOCOLATE: Maintain consumption at one serving every other day. And please remember, the serving should be half the size that it was in the previous 30 day period. Indicate, with a 0 or 1, the amount eaten today:	
CARBONATED BEVERAGES: Number of "1/2 cans" consumed today:	
COFFEE: Number of "1/2 cups" consumed today:	
ALCOHOL: Allow yourself alcoholic beverages two times every two weeks. In the space write 0, 1 or 2 corresponding to the number consumed in this two week period.	
REFINED SUGARS: Limit sugars to 1 serving and white bread to 2 servings. Enter amount consumed today:	
WATER: Drink 8 glasses of water or tea. Amount consumed today:	
EXERCISE: Walk 20 minutes without stopping. Check here when finished.	
STRETCHING EXERCISE: Do exercise Plan #3 in the back of the book. Check the box when finished.	
SLEEP: About 45 minutes before going to bed take a warm sage bath. Drink a cup of herbal tea. Read for about 20 minutes while sitting in a comfortable chair. Go to bed, lie on your back and take 3-5 deep breaths. Then work the acupressure points for sleep.	
SUPPLEMENTS: Check after taking your supplements.	
Breakfast:	
Lunch:	
Dinner:	
ON A SCALE OF 1-10, with 1 indicating symptom free and 10 indicating intense pain, rate how you feel today:	
Today's High Temperature:	

Briefly Describe Today's Weather:

What I Accomplished Today:

DAY 34

Flavored yogurt contains artificial sweeteners which are difficult for our bodies to digest. Try adding your own fruits to plain yogurt. Be sure to check that the plain yogurt you choose doesn't have artificial sweeteners in it.

CHOCOLATE: Maintain consumption at one serving every other day. And please remember, the serving should be half the size that it was in the previous 30 day period. Indicate, with a 0 or 1, the amount eaten today:	
CARBONATED BEVERAGES: Number of "1/2 cans" consumed today:	
COFFEE: Number of "1/2 cups" consumed today:	
ALCOHOL: Allow yourself alcoholic beverages two times every two weeks. In the space write 0, 1 or 2 corresponding to the number consumed in this two week period.	
REFINED SUGARS: Limit sugars to 1 serving and white bread to 2 servings. Enter amount consumed today:	
WATER: Drink 8 glasses of water or tea. Amount consumed today:	
EXERCISE: Walk 20 minutes without stopping. Check here when finished.	
STRETCHING EXERCISE: Do exercise Plan #2 in the back of the book. Check the box when finished.	
SLEEP: About 45 minutes before going to bed take a warm sage bath. Drink a cup of herbal tea. Read for about 20 minutes while sitting in a comfortable chair. Go to bed, lie on your back and take 3-5 deep breaths. Then work the acupressure points for sleep.	
SUPPLEMENTS: Check after taking your supplements.	
Breakfast:	
Lunch:	
Dinner:	
ON A SCALE OF 1-10, with 1 indicating symptom free and 10 indicating intense pain, rate how you feel today:	
Today's High Temperature:	

Briefly Describe Today's Weather:

What I Accomplished Today:

DAY 35

If you find you are craving something sweet about mid-morning and mid-afternoon, eat a piece of fruit or drink a small glass of juice or milk.

CHOCOLATE: Maintain consumption at one serving every other day. And please remember, the serving should be half the size that it was in the previous 30 day period. Indicate, with a 0 or 1, the amount eaten today:	
CARBONATED BEVERAGES: Number of "1/2 cans" consumed today:	
COFFEE: Number of "1/2 cups" consumed today:	
ALCOHOL: Allow yourself alcoholic beverages two times every two weeks. In the space write 0, 1 or 2 corresponding to the number consumed in this two week period.	
REFINED SUGARS: Limit sugars to 1 serving and white bread to 2 servings. Enter amount consumed today:	
WATER: Drink 8 glasses of water or tea. Amount consumed today:	
EXERCISE: Walk 20 minutes without stopping. Check here when finished.	
STRETCHING EXERCISE: Do exercise Plan #1 in the back of the book. Check the box when finished.	
SLEEP: About 45 minutes before going to bed take a warm sage bath. Drink a cup of herbal tea. Read for about 20 minutes while sitting in a comfortable chair. Go to bed, lie on your back and take 3-5 deep breaths. Then work the acupressure points for sleep.	
SUPPLEMENTS: Check after taking your supplements.	
Breakfast:	
Lunch:	
Dinner:	
ON A SCALE OF 1-10, with 1 indicating symptom free and 10 indicating intense pain, rate how you feel today:	
Today's High Temperature:	

Briefly Describe Today's Weather:

What I Accomplished Today:

DAY 36

Try using bananas on your cereal instead of sugar. Strawberries or other sweet fruits can also be delicious replacements for sugar.

CHOCOLATE: Maintain consumption at one serving every other day. And please remember, the serving should be half the size that it was in the previous 30 day period. Indicate, with a 0 or 1, the amount eaten today:	
CARBONATED BEVERAGES: Number of "1/2 cans" consumed today:	
COFFEE: Number of "1/2 cups" consumed today:	
ALCOHOL: Allow yourself alcoholic beverages two times every two weeks. In the space write 0, 1 or 2 corresponding to the number consumed in this two week period.	
REFINED SUGARS: Limit sugars to 1 serving and white bread to 2 servings. Enter amount consumed today:	
WATER: Drink 8 glasses of water or tea. Amount consumed today:	
EXERCISE: Walk 20 minutes without stopping. Check here when finished.	
STRETCHING EXERCISE: Do exercise Plan #2 in the back of the book. Check the box when finished.	
SLEEP: About 45 minutes before going to bed take a warm sage bath. Drink a cup of herbal tea. Read for about 20 minutes while sitting in a comfortable chair. Go to bed, lie on your back and take 3-5 deep breaths. Then work the acupressure points for sleep.	
SUPPLEMENTS: Check after taking your supplements.	
Breakfast:	
Lunch:	
Dinner:	
ON A SCALE OF 1-10, with 1 indicating symptom free and 10 indicating intense pain, rate how you feel today:	
Today's High Temperature:	

Briefly Describe Today's Weather:

What I Accomplished Today:

DAY 37

I put rolled oats into my blender and blend until it is the consistency of flour to use for my baking needs.

CHOCOLATE: Maintain consumption at one serving every other day. And please remember, the serving should be half the size that it was in the previous 30 day period. Indicate, with a 0 or 1, the amount eaten today:	
CARBONATED BEVERAGES: Number of "1/2 cans" consumed today:	
COFFEE: Number of "1/2 cups" consumed today:	
ALCOHOL: Allow yourself alcoholic beverages two times every two weeks. In the space write 0, 1 or 2 corresponding to the number consumed in this two week period.	
REFINED SUGARS: Limit sugars to 1 serving and white bread to 2 servings. Enter amount consumed today:	
WATER: Drink 8 glasses of water or tea. Amount consumed today:	
EXERCISE: Walk 20 minutes without stopping. Check here when finished.	
STRETCHING EXERCISE: Do exercise Plan #3 in the back of the book. Check the box when finished.	
SLEEP: About 45 minutes before going to bed take a warm sage bath. Drink a cup of herbal tea. Read for about 20 minutes while sitting in a comfortable chair. Go to bed, lie on your back and take 3-5 deep breaths. Then work the acupressure points for sleep.	
SUPPLEMENTS: Check after taking your supplements.	
Breakfast:	
Lunch:	
Dinner:	
ON A SCALE OF 1-10, with 1 indicating symptom free and 10 indicating intense pain, rate how you feel today:	
Today's High Temperature:	

Briefly Describe Today's Weather:

What I Accomplished Today:

DAY 38

Flour tortilla shells make great low-fat pie crusts! Just put them in the pie pan before the fruit.

CHOCOLATE: Maintain consumption at one serving every other day. And please remember, the serving should be half the size that it was in the previous 30 day period. Indicate, with a 0 or 1, the amount eaten today:	
CARBONATED BEVERAGES: Number of "1/2 cans" consumed today:	
COFFEE: Number of "1/2 cups" consumed today:	
ALCOHOL: Allow yourself alcoholic beverages two times every two weeks. In the space write 0, 1 or 2 corresponding to the number consumed in this two week period.	
REFINED SUGARS: Limit sugars to 1 serving and white bread to 2 servings. Enter amount consumed today:	
WATER: Drink 8 glasses of water or tea. Amount consumed today:	
EXERCISE: Walk 20 minutes without stopping. Check here when finished.	
STRETCHING EXERCISE: Do exercise Plan #1 in the back of the book. Check the box when finished.	
SLEEP: About 45 minutes before going to bed take a warm sage bath. Drink a cup of herbal tea. Read for about 20 minutes while sitting in a comfortable chair. Go to bed, lie on your back and take 3-5 deep breaths. Then work the acupressure points for sleep.	
SUPPLEMENTS: Check after taking your supplements.	
Breakfast:	
Lunch:	
Dinner:	
ON A SCALE OF 1-10, with 1 indicating symptom free and 10 indicating intense pain, rate how you feel today:	
Today's High Temperature:	

Briefly Describe Today's Weather:

What I Accomplished Today:

DAY 39

When making burritos, try using beans (red, white, navy, or any kind) in place of meat. Delicious, nutritious and low in fat!

CHOCOLATE: Maintain consumption at one serving every other day. And please remember, the serving should be half the size that it was in the previous 30 day period. Indicate, with a 0 or 1, the amount eaten today:	
CARBONATED BEVERAGES: Number of "1/2 cans" consumed today:	
COFFEE: Number of "1/2 cups" consumed today:	
ALCOHOL: Allow yourself alcoholic beverages two times every two weeks. In the space write 0, 1 or 2 corresponding to the number consumed in this two week period.	
REFINED SUGARS: Limit sugars to 1 serving and white bread to 2 servings. Enter amount consumed today:	
WATER: Drink 8 glasses of water or tea. Amount consumed today:	
EXERCISE: Walk 20 minutes without stopping. Check here when finished.	
STRETCHING EXERCISE: Do exercise Plan #2 in the back of the book. Check the box when finished.	
SLEEP: About 45 minutes before going to bed take a warm sage bath. Drink a cup of herbal tea. Read for about 20 minutes while sitting in a comfortable chair. Go to bed, lie on your back and take 3-5 deep breaths. Then work the acupressure points for sleep.	
SUPPLEMENTS: Check after taking your supplements.	
Breakfast:	
Lunch:	
Dinner:	
ON A SCALE OF 1-10, with 1 indicating symptom free and 10 indicating intense pain, rate how you feel today:	
Today's High Temperature:	

Briefly Describe Today's Weather:

What I Accomplished Today:

DAY 40

Flaxseed is very inexpensive and full of both essential fatty acids and fiber. I add flaxseed to my cereals, milk shakes and breakfast drinks.

CHOCOLATE: Maintain consumption at one serving every other day. And please remember, the serving should be half the size that it was in the previous 30 day period. Indicate, with a 0 or 1, the amount eaten today:	
CARBONATED BEVERAGES: Number of "1/2 cans" consumed today:	
COFFEE: Number of "1/2 cups" consumed today:	
ALCOHOL: Allow yourself alcoholic beverages two times every two weeks. In the space write 0, 1 or 2 corresponding to the number consumed in this two week period.	
REFINED SUGARS: Limit sugars to 1 serving and white bread to 2 servings. Enter amount consumed today:	
WATER: Drink 8 glasses of water or tea. Amount consumed today:	
EXERCISE: Walk 20 minutes without stopping. Check here when finished.	
STRETCHING EXERCISE: Do exercise Plan #3 in the back of the book. Check the box when finished.	
SLEEP: About 45 minutes before going to bed take a warm sage bath. Drink a cup of herbal tea. Read for about 20 minutes while sitting in a comfortable chair. Go to bed, lie on your back and take 3-5 deep breaths. Then work the acupressure points for sleep.	
SUPPLEMENTS: Check after taking your supplements.	
Breakfast:	
Lunch:	
Dinner:	
ON A SCALE OF 1-10, with 1 indicating symptom free and 10 indicating intense pain, rate how you feel today:	
Today's High Temperature:	

Briefly Describe Today's Weather:

What I Accomplished Today:

DAY 41

Many people have noticed reduced pain after taking flaxseed over a period of a few weeks.

CHOCOLATE: Maintain consumption at one serving every other day. And please remember, the serving should be half the size that it was in the previous 30 day period. Indicate, with a 0 or 1, the amount eaten today:	
CARBONATED BEVERAGES: Number of "1/2 cans" consumed today:	
COFFEE: Number of "1/2 cups" consumed today:	
ALCOHOL: Allow yourself alcoholic beverages two times every two weeks. In the space write 0, 1 or 2 corresponding to the number consumed in this two week period.	
REFINED SUGARS: Limit sugars to 1 serving and white bread to 2 servings. Enter amount consumed today:	
WATER: Drink 8 glasses of water or tea. Amount consumed today:	
EXERCISE: Walk 20 minutes without stopping. Check here when finished.	
STRETCHING EXERCISE: Do exercise Plan #1 in the back of the book. Check the box when finished.	
SLEEP: About 45 minutes before going to bed take a warm sage bath. Drink a cup of herbal tea. Read for about 20 minutes while sitting in a comfortable chair. Go to bed, lie on your back and take 3-5 deep breaths. Then work the acupressure points for sleep.	
SUPPLEMENTS: Check after taking your supplements.	
Breakfast:	
Lunch:	
Dinner:	
ON A SCALE OF 1-10, with 1 indicating symptom free and 10 indicating intense pain, rate how you feel today:	
Today's High Temperature:	

Briefly Describe Today's Weather:

What I Accomplished Today:

DAY 42

To make my life easier, and to keep cooking down to a minimum, I try to make double of the servings of food my family will eat in a typical meal. Then I freeze the extra to be used at another time.

CHOCOLATE: Maintain consumption at one serving every other day. And please remember, the serving should be half the size that it was in the previous 30 day period. Indicate, with a 0 or 1, the amount eaten today:	
CARBONATED BEVERAGES: Number of "1/2 cans" consumed today:	
COFFEE: Number of "1/2 cups" consumed today:	
ALCOHOL: Allow yourself alcoholic beverages two times every two weeks. In the space write 0, 1 or 2 corresponding to the number consumed in this two week period.	
REFINED SUGARS: Limit sugars to 1 serving and white bread to 2 servings. Enter amount consumed today:	
WATER: Drink 8 glasses of water or tea. Amount consumed today:	
EXERCISE: Walk 20 minutes without stopping. Check here when finished.	
STRETCHING EXERCISE: Do exercise Plan #2 in the back of the book. Check the box when finished.	
SLEEP: About 45 minutes before going to bed take a warm sage bath. Drink a cup of herbal tea. Read for about 20 minutes while sitting in a comfortable chair. Go to bed, lie on your back and take 3-5 deep breaths. Then work the acupressure points for sleep.	
SUPPLEMENTS: Check after taking your supplements.	
Breakfast:	
Lunch:	
Dinner:	
ON A SCALE OF 1-10, with 1 indicating symptom free and 10 indicating intense pain, rate how you feel today:	
Today's High Temperature:	

Briefly Describe Today's Weather:

What I Accomplished Today:

DAY 43

Parsley is very easy to grow and requires little care. One handful of parsley per day can provide many essential nutrients and is a good source of calcium. To dry parsley, hang it upside down in a paper bag in a dark room or closet.

CHOCOLATE: Maintain consumption at one serving every other day. The serving should be half the size that it was in the previous 30 day period. Indicate, with a 0 or 1, the amount eaten today:	
CARBONATED BEVERAGES: Number of "1/2 cans" consumed today:	
COFFEE: Number of "1/2 cups" consumed today:	
ALCOHOL: Allow yourself alcoholic beverages two times every two weeks. In the space write 0, 1 or 2 corresponding to the number consumed in this two week period.	
REFINED SUGARS: Limit sugars to 1 serving and white bread to 2 servings. Enter amount consumed today:	
WATER: Drink 8 glasses of water or tea. Amount consumed today:	
EXERCISE: Walk 20 minutes without stopping. Check here when finished.	
STRETCHING EXERCISE: Do exercise Plan #3 in the back of the book. Check the box when finished.	
SLEEP: About 45 minutes before going to bed take a warm sage bath. Drink a cup of herbal tea. Read for about 20 minutes while sitting in a comfortable chair. Go to bed, lie on your back and take 3-5 deep breaths. Then work the acupressure points for sleep.	
SUPPLEMENTS: Check after taking your supplements.	
Breakfast:	
Lunch:	
Dinner:	
ON A SCALE OF 1-10, with 1 indicating symptom free and 10 indicating intense pain, rate how you feel today:	
Today's High Temperature:	

Briefly Describe Today's Weather:

What I Accomplished Today:

DAY 44

Sage is another perennial herb which requires little care, yet it has so many wonderful uses. Dry as described for parsley. (Day 43)

CHOCOLATE: Maintain consumption at one serving every other day. The serving should be half the size that it was in the previous 30 day period. Indicate, with a 0 or 1, the amount eaten today:	
CARBONATED BEVERAGES: Number of "1/2 cans" consumed today:	
COFFEE: Number of "1/2 cups" consumed today:	
ALCOHOL: Allow yourself alcoholic beverages two times every two weeks. In the space write 0, 1 or 2 corresponding to the number consumed in this two week period.	
REFINED SUGARS: Limit sugars to 1 serving and white bread to 2 servings. Enter amount consumed today:	
WATER: Drink 8 glasses of water or tea. Amount consumed today:	
EXERCISE: Walk 20 minutes without stopping. Check here when finished.	
STRETCHING EXERCISE: Do exercise Plan #1 in the back of the book. Check the box when finished.	
SLEEP: About 45 minutes before going to bed take a warm sage bath. Drink a cup of herbal tea. Read for about 20 minutes while sitting in a comfortable chair. Go to bed, lie on your back and take 3-5 deep breaths. Then work the acupressure points for sleep.	
SUPPLEMENTS: Check after taking your supplements.	
Breakfast:	
Lunch:	
Dinner:	
ON A SCALE OF 1-10, with 1 indicating symptom free and 10 indicating intense pain, rate how you feel today:	
Today's High Temperature:	

Briefly Describe Today's Weather:

What I Accomplished Today:

DAY 45

Mint does wonders for an upset stomach.

CHOCOLATE: Maintain consumption at one serving every other day. The serving should be half the size that it was in the previous 30 day period. Indicate, with a 0 or 1, the amount eaten today:	
CARBONATED BEVERAGES: Number of "1/2 cans" consumed today:	
COFFEE: Number of "1/2 cups" consumed today:	
ALCOHOL: Allow yourself alcoholic beverages two times every two weeks. In the space write 0, 1 or 2 corresponding to the number consumed in this two week period.	
REFINED SUGARS: Limit sugars to 1 serving and white bread to 2 servings. Enter amount consumed today:	
WATER: Drink 8 glasses of water or tea. Amount consumed today:	
EXERCISE: Walk 20 minutes without stopping. Check here when finished.	
STRETCHING EXERCISE: Do exercise Plan #2 in the back of the book. Check the box when finished.	
SLEEP: About 45 minutes before going to bed take a warm sage bath. Drink a cup of herbal tea. Read for about 20 minutes while sitting in a comfortable chair. Go to bed, lie on your back and take 3-5 deep breaths. Then work the acupressure points for sleep.	
SUPPLEMENTS: Check after taking your supplements.	
Breakfast:	
Lunch:	
Dinner:	
ON A SCALE OF 1-10, with 1 indicating symptom free and 10 indicating intense pain, rate how you feel today:	
Today's High Temperature:	

Briefly Describe Today's Weather:

What I Accomplished Today:

DAY 46

Mint plants make a pleasant addition to any garden. Be sure to plant them where they have plenty of room to spread.

CHOCOLATE: Maintain consumption at one serving every other day. The serving should be half the size that it was in the previous 30 day period. Indicate, with a 0 or 1, the amount eaten today:	
CARBONATED BEVERAGES: Number of "1/2 cans" consumed today:	
COFFEE: Number of "1/2 cups" consumed today:	
ALCOHOL: Allow yourself alcoholic beverages two times every two weeks. In the space write 0, 1 or 2 corresponding to the number consumed in this two week period.	
REFINED SUGARS: Limit sugars to 1 serving and white bread to 2 servings. Enter amount consumed today:	
WATER: Drink 8 glasses of water or tea. Amount consumed today:	
EXERCISE: Walk 20 minutes without stopping. Check here when finished.	
STRETCHING EXERCISE: Do exercise Plan #3 in the back of the book. Check the box when finished.	
SLEEP: About 45 minutes before going to bed take a warm sage bath. Drink a cup of herbal tea. Read for about 20 minutes while sitting in a comfortable chair. Go to bed, lie on your back and take 3-5 deep breaths. Then work the acupressure points for sleep.	
SUPPLEMENTS: Check after taking your supplements.	
Breakfast:	
Lunch:	
Dinner:	
ON A SCALE OF 1-10, with 1 indicating symptom free and 10 indicating intense pain, rate how you feel today:	
Today's High Temperature:	

Briefly Describe Today's Weather:

What I Accomplished Today:

DAY 47

A strong peppermint tea can help ward off a cold when taken as soon as symptoms appear.

CHOCOLATE: Maintain consumption at one serving every other day. The serving should be half the size that it was in the previous 30 day period. Indicate, with a 0 or 1, the amount eaten today:	
CARBONATED BEVERAGES: Number of "1/2 cans" consumed today:	
COFFEE: Number of "1/2 cups" consumed today:	
ALCOHOL: Allow yourself alcoholic beverages two times every two weeks. In the space write 0, 1 or 2 corresponding to the number consumed in this two week period.	
REFINED SUGARS: Limit sugars to 1 serving and white bread to 2 servings. Enter amount consumed today:	
WATER: Drink 8 glasses of water or tea. Amount consumed today:	
EXERCISE: Walk 20 minutes without stopping. Check here when finished.	
STRETCHING EXERCISE: Do exercise Plan #3 in the back of the book. Check the box when finished.	
SLEEP: About 45 minutes before going to bed take a warm sage bath. Drink a cup of herbal tea. Read for about 20 minutes while sitting in a comfortable chair. Go to bed, lie on your back and take 3-5 deep breaths. Then work the acupressure points for sleep.	
SUPPLEMENTS: Check after taking your supplements.	
Breakfast:	
Lunch:	
Dinner:	
ON A SCALE OF 1-10, with 1 indicating symptom free and 10 indicating intense pain, rate how you feel today:	
Today's High Temperature:	

Briefly Describe Today's Weather:

What I Accomplished Today:

DAY 48

Rubbing mint leaves on the forehead and temples is said to help relieve headaches. Plus, you might say that it "leaves" you smelling "minty fresh."

CHOCOLATE: Maintain consumption at one serving every other day. The serving should be half the size that it was in the previous 30 day period. Indicate, with a 0 or 1, the amount eaten today:	
CARBONATED BEVERAGES: Number of "1/2 cans" consumed today:	
COFFEE: Number of "1/2 cups" consumed today:	
ALCOHOL: Allow yourself alcoholic beverages two times every two weeks. In the space write 0, 1 or 2 corresponding to the number consumed in this two week period.	
REFINED SUGARS: Limit sugars to 1 serving and white bread to 2 servings. Enter amount consumed today:	
WATER: Drink 8 glasses of water or tea. Amount consumed today:	
EXERCISE: Walk 20 minutes without stopping. Check here when finished.	
STRETCHING EXERCISE: Do exercise Plan #1 in the back of the book. Check the box when finished.	
SLEEP: About 45 minutes before going to bed take a warm sage bath. Drink a cup of herbal tea. Read for about 20 minutes while sitting in a comfortable chair. Go to bed, lie on your back and take 3-5 deep breaths. Then work the acupressure points for sleep.	
SUPPLEMENTS: Check after taking your supplements.	
Breakfast:	
Lunch:	
Dinner:	
ON A SCALE OF 1-10, with 1 indicating symptom free and 10 indicating intense pain, rate how you feel today:	
Today's High Temperature:	

Briefly Describe Today's Weather:

What I Accomplished Today:

DAY 49

Chamomile likes to be placed in an area where it will be stepped on. When mixed with mint and catnip and consumed as a tea, it is an excellent way to help to get a good night's sleep.

CHOCOLATE: Maintain consumption at one serving every other day. The serving should be half the size that it was in the previous 30 day period. Indicate, with a 0 or 1, the amount eaten today:	
CARBONATED BEVERAGES: Number of "1/2 cans" consumed today:	
COFFEE: Number of "1/2 cups" consumed today:	
ALCOHOL: Allow yourself alcoholic beverages two times every two weeks. In the space write 0, 1 or 2 corresponding to the number consumed in this two week period.	
REFINED SUGARS: Limit sugars to 1 serving and white bread to 2 servings. Enter amount consumed today:	
WATER: Drink 8 glasses of water or tea. Amount consumed today:	
EXERCISE: Walk 20 minutes without stopping. Check here when finished.	
STRETCHING EXERCISE: Do exercise Plan #2 in the back of the book. Check the box when finished.	
SLEEP: About 45 minutes before going to bed take a warm sage bath. Drink a cup of herbal tea. Read for about 20 minutes while sitting in a comfortable chair. Go to bed, lie on your back and take 3-5 deep breaths. Then work the acupressure points for sleep.	
SUPPLEMENTS: Check after taking your supplements.	
Breakfast:	
Lunch:	
Dinner:	
ON A SCALE OF 1-10, with 1 indicating symptom free and 10 indicating intense pain, rate how you feel today:	
Today's High Temperature:	

Briefly Describe Today's Weather:

What I Accomplished Today:

DAY 50

Catnip is wonderful for relaxation and is a good source of vitamin C. When mixed with chamomile and mint and taken as a tea, it is an excellent way to help get a good night's sleep.

CHOCOLATE: Maintain consumption at one serving every other day. The serving should be half the size that it was in the previous 30 day period. Indicate, with a 0 or 1, the amount eaten today:	
CARBONATED BEVERAGES: Number of "1/2 cans" consumed today:	
COFFEE: Number of "1/2 cups" consumed today:	
ALCOHOL: Allow yourself alcoholic beverages two times every two weeks. In the space write 0, 1 or 2 corresponding to the number consumed in this two week period.	
REFINED SUGARS: Limit sugars to 1 serving and white bread to 2 servings. Enter amount consumed today:	
WATER: Drink 8 glasses of water or tea. Amount consumed today:	
EXERCISE: Walk 20 minutes without stopping. Check here when finished.	
STRETCHING EXERCISE: Do exercise Plan #3 in the back of the book. Check the box when finished.	
SLEEP: About 45 minutes before going to bed take a warm sage bath. Drink a cup of herbal tea. Read for about 20 minutes while sitting in a comfortable chair. Go to bed, lie on your back and take 3-5 deep breaths. Then work the acupressure points for sleep.	
SUPPLEMENTS: Check after taking your supplements.	
Breakfast:	
Lunch:	
Dinner:	
ON A SCALE OF 1-10, with 1 indicating symptom free and 10 indicating intense pain, rate how you feel today:	
Today's High Temperature:	

Briefly Describe Today's Weather:

What I Accomplished Today:

DAY 51

Catnip tea also helps reduce flatulence. (And that can be a relief to those around you as well!)

CHOCOLATE: Maintain consumption at one serving every other day. The serving should be half the size that it was in the previous 30 day period. Indicate, with a 0 or 1, the amount eaten today:	
CARBONATED BEVERAGES: Number of "1/2 cans" consumed today:	
COFFEE: Number of "1/2 cups" consumed today:	
ALCOHOL: Allow yourself alcoholic beverages two times every two weeks. In the space write 0, 1 or 2 corresponding to the number consumed in this two week period.	
REFINED SUGARS: Limit sugars to 1 serving and white bread to 2 servings. Enter amount consumed today:	
WATER: Drink 8 glasses of water or tea. Amount consumed today:	
EXERCISE: Walk 20 minutes without stopping. Check here when finished.	
STRETCHING EXERCISE: Do exercise Plan #3 in the back of the book. Check the box when finished.	
SLEEP: About 45 minutes before going to bed take a warm sage bath. Drink a cup of herbal tea. Read for about 20 minutes while sitting in a comfortable chair. Go to bed, lie on your back and take 3-5 deep breaths. Then work the acupressure points for sleep.	
SUPPLEMENTS: Check after taking your supplements.	
Breakfast:	
Lunch:	
Dinner:	
ON A SCALE OF 1-10, with 1 indicating symptom free and 10 indicating intense pain, rate how you feel today:	
Today's High Temperature:	

Briefly Describe Today's Weather:

What I Accomplished Today:

DAY 52

Recently while talking to some women who had attended one of my programs the question was asked: "Do you really feel as good as you say you do?" My answer: "I feel better than I have in more than 20 years."

CHOCOLATE: Maintain consumption at one serving every other day. The serving should be half the size that it was in the previous 30 day period. Indicate, with a 0 or 1, the amount eaten today:	
CARBONATED BEVERAGES: Number of "1/2 cans" consumed today:	
COFFEE: Number of "1/2 cups" consumed today:	
ALCOHOL: Allow yourself alcoholic beverages two times every two weeks. In the space write 0, 1 or 2 corresponding to the number consumed in this two week period.	
REFINED SUGARS: Limit sugars to 1 serving and white bread to 2 servings. Enter amount consumed today:	
WATER: Drink 8 glasses of water or tea. Amount consumed today:	
EXERCISE: Walk 20 minutes without stopping. Check here when finished.	
STRETCHING EXERCISE: Do exercise Plan #1 in the back of the book. Check the box when finished.	
SLEEP: About 45 minutes before going to bed take a warm sage bath. Drink a cup of herbal tea. Read for about 20 minutes while sitting in a comfortable chair. Go to bed, lie on your back and take 3-5 deep breaths. Then work the acupressure points for sleep.	
SUPPLEMENTS: Check after taking your supplements.	
Breakfast:	
Lunch:	
Dinner:	
ON A SCALE OF 1-10, with 1 indicating symptom free and 10 indicating intense pain, rate how you feel today:	
Today's High Temperature:	

Briefly Describe Today's Weather:

What I Accomplished Today:

DAY 53

For years I thought everyone woke up every morning feeling like they had been beaten up during the night. I couldn't believe how wrong I was!

CHOCOLATE: Maintain consumption at one serving every other day. The serving should be half the size that it was in the previous 30 day period. Indicate, with a 0 or 1, the amount eaten today:	
CARBONATED BEVERAGES: Number of "1/2 cans" consumed today:	
COFFEE: Number of "1/2 cups" consumed today:	
ALCOHOL: Allow yourself alcoholic beverages two times every two weeks. In the space write 0, 1 or 2 corresponding to the number consumed in this two week period.	
REFINED SUGARS: Limit sugars to 1 serving and white bread to 2 servings. Enter amount consumed today:	
WATER: Drink 8 glasses of water or tea. Amount consumed today:	
EXERCISE: Walk 20 minutes without stopping. Check here when finished.	
STRETCHING EXERCISE: Do exercise Plan #1 in the back of the book. Check the box when finished.	
SLEEP: About 45 minutes before going to bed take a warm sage bath. Drink a cup of herbal tea. Read for about 20 minutes while sitting in a comfortable chair. Go to bed, lie on your back and take 3-5 deep breaths. Then work the acupressure points for sleep.	
SUPPLEMENTS: Check after taking your supplements.	
Breakfast:	
Lunch:	
Dinner:	
ON A SCALE OF 1-10, with 1 indicating symptom free and 10 indicating intense pain, rate how you feel today:	
Today's High Temperature:	

Briefly Describe Today's Weather:

What I Accomplished Today:

DAY 54

With our bodies working less efficiently, toxins aren't released properly. It is believed this causes a toxic buildup in the tissues, which can also cause pain.

CHOCOLATE: Maintain consumption at one serving every other day. The serving should be half the size that it was in the previous 30 day period. Indicate, with a 0 or 1, the amount eaten today:	
CARBONATED BEVERAGES: Number of "1/2 cans" consumed today:	
COFFEE: Number of "1/2 cups" consumed today:	
ALCOHOL: Allow yourself alcoholic beverages two times every two weeks. In the space write 0, 1 or 2 corresponding to the number consumed in this two week period.	
REFINED SUGARS: Limit sugars to 1 serving and white bread to 2 servings. Enter amount consumed today:	
WATER: Drink 8 glasses of water or tea. Amount consumed today:	
EXERCISE: Walk 20 minutes without stopping. Check here when finished.	
STRETCHING EXERCISE: Do exercise Plan #2 in the back of the book. Check the box when finished.	
SLEEP: About 45 minutes before going to bed take a warm sage bath. Drink a cup of herbal tea. Read for about 20 minutes while sitting in a comfortable chair. Go to bed, lie on your back and take 3-5 deep breaths. Then work the acupressure points for sleep.	
SUPPLEMENTS: Check after taking your supplements.	
Breakfast:	
Lunch:	
Dinner:	
ON A SCALE OF 1-10, with 1 indicating symptom free and 10 indicating intense pain, rate how you feel today:	
Today's High Temperature:	

Briefly Describe Today's Weather:

What I Accomplished Today:

DAY 55

Tight muscles can also create pain. If you notice tension or pain increasing in an area of your body, gently stretch that area.

CHOCOLATE: Maintain consumption at one serving every other day. The serving should be half the size that it was in the previous 30 day period. Indicate, with a 0 or 1, the amount eaten today:	
CARBONATED BEVERAGES: Number of "1/2 cans" consumed today:	
COFFEE: Number of "1/2 cups" consumed today:	
ALCOHOL: Allow yourself alcoholic beverages two times every two weeks. In the space write 0, 1 or 2 corresponding to the number consumed in this two week period.	
REFINED SUGARS: Limit sugars to 1 serving and white bread to 2 servings. Enter amount consumed today:	
WATER: Drink 8 glasses of water or tea. Amount consumed today:	
EXERCISE: Walk 20 minutes without stopping. Check here when finished.	
STRETCHING EXERCISE: Do exercise Plan #3 in the back of the book. Check the box when finished.	
SLEEP: About 45 minutes before going to bed take a warm sage bath. Drink a cup of herbal tea. Read for about 20 minutes while sitting in a comfortable chair. Go to bed, lie on your back and take 3-5 deep breaths. Then work the acupressure points for sleep.	
SUPPLEMENTS: Check after taking your supplements.	
Breakfast:	
Lunch:	
Dinner:	
ON A SCALE OF 1-10, with 1 indicating symptom free and 10 indicating intense pain, rate how you feel today:	
Today's High Temperature:	

Briefly Describe Today's Weather:

What I Accomplished Today:

DAY 56

Many times pain in the back of the head can be reduced by massaging around the occipital bone at the lower base of the skull in the back of the head.

CHOCOLATE: Maintain consumption at one serving every other day. The serving should be half the size that it was in the previous 30 day period. Indicate, with a 0 or 1, the amount eaten today:	
CARBONATED BEVERAGES: Number of "1/2 cans" consumed today:	
COFFEE: Number of "1/2 cups" consumed today:	
ALCOHOL: Allow yourself alcoholic beverages two times every two weeks. In the space write 0, 1 or 2 corresponding to the number consumed in this two week period.	
REFINED SUGARS: Limit sugars to 1 serving and white bread to 2 servings. Enter amount consumed today:	
WATER: Drink 8 glasses of water or tea. Amount consumed today:	
EXERCISE: Walk 20 minutes without stopping. Check here when finished.	
STRETCHING EXERCISE: Do exercise Plan #1 in the back of the book. Check the box when finished.	
SLEEP: About 45 minutes before going to bed take a warm sage bath. Drink a cup of herbal tea. Read for about 20 minutes while sitting in a comfortable chair. Go to bed, lie on your back and take 3-5 deep breaths. Then work the acupressure points for sleep.	
SUPPLEMENTS: Check after taking your supplements.	
Breakfast:	
Lunch:	
Dinner:	
ON A SCALE OF 1-10, with 1 indicating symptom free and 10 indicating intense pain, rate how you feel today:	
Today's High Temperature:	

Briefly Describe Today's Weather:

What I Accomplished Today:

DAY 57

It is believed by some that the areas of pain around the base of the occipital area in the head are related to organs within the body that are stressed.

CHOCOLATE: Maintain consumption at one serving every other day. The serving should be half the size that it was in the previous 30 day period. Indicate, with a 0 or 1, the amount eaten today:	
CARBONATED BEVERAGES: Number of "1/2 cans" consumed today:	
COFFEE: Number of "1/2 cups" consumed today:	
ALCOHOL: Allow yourself alcoholic beverages two times every two weeks. In the space write 0, 1 or 2 corresponding to the number consumed in this two week period.	
REFINED SUGARS: Limit sugars to 1 serving and white bread to 2 servings. Enter amount consumed today:	
WATER: Drink 8 glasses of water or tea. Amount consumed today:	
EXERCISE: Walk 20 minutes without stopping. Check here when finished.	
STRETCHING EXERCISE: Do exercise Plan #1 in the back of the book. Check the box when finished.	
SLEEP: About 45 minutes before going to bed take a warm sage bath. Drink a cup of herbal tea. Read for about 20 minutes while sitting in a comfortable chair. Go to bed, lie on your back and take 3-5 deep breaths. Then work the acupressure points for sleep.	
SUPPLEMENTS: Check after taking your supplements.	
Breakfast:	
Lunch:	
Dinner:	
ON A SCALE OF 1-10, with 1 indicating symptom free and 10 indicating intense pain, rate how you feel today:	
Today's High Temperature:	

Briefly Describe Today's Weather:

What I Accomplished Today:

DAY 58

Our bodies need the proper food or "fuel" to run smoothly. If we put something other than gasoline into the gas tank of our car, we all know what happens.

CHOCOLATE: Maintain consumption at one serving every other day. The serving should be half the size that it was in the previous 30 day period. Indicate, with a 0 or 1, the amount eaten today:	
CARBONATED BEVERAGES: Number of "1/2 cans" consumed today:	
COFFEE: Number of "1/2 cups" consumed today:	
ALCOHOL: Allow yourself alcoholic beverages two times every two weeks. In the space write 0, 1 or 2 corresponding to the number consumed in this two week period.	
REFINED SUGARS: Limit sugars to 1 serving and white bread to 2 servings. Enter amount consumed today:	
WATER: Drink 8 glasses of water or tea. Amount consumed today:	
EXERCISE: Walk 20 minutes without stopping. Check here when finished.	
STRETCHING EXERCISE: Do exercise Plan #2 in the back of the book. Check the box when finished.	
SLEEP: About 45 minutes before going to bed take a warm sage bath. Drink a cup of herbal tea. Read for about 20 minutes while sitting in a comfortable chair. Go to bed, lie on your back and take 3-5 deep breaths. Then work the acupressure points for sleep.	
SUPPLEMENTS: Check after taking your supplements.	
Breakfast:	
Lunch:	
Dinner:	
ON A SCALE OF 1-10, with 1 indicating symptom free and 10 indicating intense pain, rate how you feel today:	
Today's High Temperature:	

Briefly Describe Today's Weather:

What I Accomplished Today:

DAY 59

Can you believe you have almost made it to the 60 day mark? By now you should be well into the program. Keep up the good work.

CHOCOLATE: Maintain consumption at one serving every other day. The serving should be half the size that it was in the previous 30 day period. Indicate, with a 0 or 1, the amount eaten today:	
CARBONATED BEVERAGES: Number of "1/2 cans" consumed today:	
COFFEE: Number of "1/2 cups" consumed today:	
ALCOHOL: Allow yourself alcoholic beverages two times every two weeks. In the space write 0, 1 or 2 corresponding to the number consumed in this two week period.	
REFINED SUGARS: Limit sugars to 1 serving and white bread to 2 servings. Enter amount consumed today:	
WATER: Drink 8 glasses of water or tea. Amount consumed today:	
EXERCISE: Walk 20 minutes without stopping. Check here when finished.	
STRETCHING EXERCISE: Do exercise Plan #3 in the back of the book. Check the box when finished.	
SLEEP: About 45 minutes before going to bed take a warm sage bath. Drink a cup of herbal tea. Read for about 20 minutes while sitting in a comfortable chair. Go to bed, lie on your back and take 3-5 deep breaths. Then work the acupressure points for sleep.	
SUPPLEMENTS: Check after taking your supplements.	
Breakfast:	
Lunch:	
Dinner:	
ON A SCALE OF 1-10, with 1 indicating symptom free and 10 indicating intense pain, rate how you feel today:	
Today's High Temperature:	

Briefly Describe Today's Weather:

What I Accomplished Today:

DAY 60

Congratulations! You've made it through 60 days. From here on it should get easier. You have been making some drastic changes in your lifestyle. Keep working, because you'll be glad you did.

CHOCOLATE: Maintain consumption at one serving every other day. The serving should be half the size that it was in the previous 30 day period. Indicate, with a 0 or 1, the amount eaten today:	
CARBONATED BEVERAGES: Number of "1/2 cans" consumed today:	
COFFEE: Number of "1/2 cups" consumed today:	
ALCOHOL: Allow yourself alcoholic beverages two times every two weeks. In the space write 0, 1 or 2 corresponding to the number consumed in this two week period.	
REFINED SUGARS: Limit sugars to 1 serving and white bread to 2 servings. Enter amount consumed today:	
WATER: Drink 8 glasses of water or tea. Amount consumed today:	
EXERCISE: Walk 20 minutes without stopping. Check here when finished.	
STRETCHING EXERCISE: Do exercise Plan #1 in the back of the book. Check the box when finished.	
SLEEP: About 45 minutes before going to bed take a warm sage bath. Drink a cup of herbal tea. Read for about 20 minutes while sitting in a comfortable chair. Go to bed, lie on your back and take 3-5 deep breaths. Then work the acupressure points for sleep.	
SUPPLEMENTS: Check after taking your supplements.	
Breakfast:	
Lunch:	
Dinner:	
ON A SCALE OF 1-10, with 1 indicating symptom free and 10 indicating intense pain, rate how you feel today:	
Today's High Temperature:	

Briefly Describe Today's Weather:

What I Accomplished Today:

HEALTH EVALUATION FORM

Indicate in the column next to the symptoms which of the following conditions apply to you in terms of frequency and/or intensity of symptoms using the numbers of 1-10: With 1 indicating the least and 10 indicating the greatest intensity or frequency.

Low Energy	____	Often Feel Tired	____	Headaches	____
Dry/itchy Skin	____	Dry or Itchy scalp	____	Rashes or Eczema	____
Achy Joints	____	Muscle Cramps	____	Muscle Twitches	____
Bruising	____	Menstrual Cramps	____	Moody/PMS	____
Poor Concentration	__	Water Retention	____	Bowel Gas	____
Numbing/Tingling	____	Skin Burning	____	Dry Eyes	____
Weak Fingernails	____	Dry/Brittle Hair	____	Weak Muscles	____
Joint Pain	____	Foot Pain	____	TMJ Pain	____

Indigestion/Acid Reflux	____	Constipation and/or Diarrhea	____
Frequently Take Pain Killers	____	Difficulty Handling Stress	____
High/Low Blood Pressure	____	Strong Desire for Sweets/Salts	____
Moods of Depression	____	Often feel Bloated	____
Cold Hands and Feet	____	Difficulty Falling Asleep	____
Shortness of Breath	____	Allergies and/or Hayfever	____
Poor Night Vision	____	Light Sleep/Aware of Surroundings	____

NOTE: Once you have completed this health evaluation, return to the first health evaluation and second evaluation to compare the improvements. Remember, improvement will be gradual. By filling out the health evaluation monthly it will be easier to continue to see the progress your body is making during its healing process.

Now, get ready to live! Here comes the third, 30 day period.

The Miracle

I saw a miracle today
As I was walking by.
Not on the ground or in the water
But rather, in the sky.
And as I watched this miracle
My heart would leap in joy;
That such a wonder could come my way,
In the middle of the day.
This miracle high up in the sky
Was playing like a child.
Actually not one or two or three or four
But many birds, from the wild.
As they flew up in the distance
And turned and whirled and traveled;
Their wings would glisten and disappear,
then turn black as the picture unraveled.
This wonderful miracle I watched in awe
For a very short time that day;
Enjoying nature's gift to me
As in their world they played.
Then as quickly as they came, they also disappeared.
On their way to who knows where
As the sky I watched was cleared
I thank the earth for her gifts of beauty;
And I am thankful for this day.
I'm thankful for the flock of birds
And the ability to watch them play
The lesson nature taught me today by this beautiful show.
Is to stop and watch and enjoy each thing
As on our paths we go.

Mary Moeller

DAY 61

We will make a few more changes this month, so be sure to read through each area carefully.

CHOCOLATE: Allow one serving, twice a week. Note the amount eaten today:	
CARBONATED BEVERAGES: Beginning today you will only drink one "1/2 can," 3 times a week. Write 0 to indicate if you consumed no cans, or 1,2 or 3 for the first, second, or third "1/2 can" this week.	
COFFEE: Beginning today you will only drink one "1/2 cup" 3 times a week. Write 0 to indicate if you did not have any cups, or 1,2 or 3 for the first, second, or third cup this week.	
ALCOHOL: Allow no more than two drinks over the course of the next 30 days. In the space indicate the first and second drink. Write in a 0 for all the days in which you do not imbibe.	
REFINED SUGARS: Limit sugar consumption to once every other day and white bread to 2 servings a day. Enter number of servings consumed:	
WATER: Drink 8 glasses of water. Amount consumed today:	
EXERCISE: Walk briskly for 30 minutes without stopping. Check here when finished.	
STRETCHING: Do exercise Plan #1. Check here when finished.	
SLEEP: Utilize ideas from "Natural Sleep Aids" chapter.	
SUPPLEMENTS: Check here after taking your supplements.	
Breakfast:	
Lunch:	
Dinner:	
ON A SCALE OF 1-10, with 1 indicating that you are free of symptoms, rate how you feel today:	
Today's High Temperature:	

Briefly Describe Today's Weather:

What I Accomplished Today:

DAY 62

Okay, so you're getting a little tired of this old drag of watching everything that goes into your mouth. I know the feeling, but don't forget that most of us who feel good have been through it. Remember, you can drink a small glass of juice or eat a small piece of fruit every two hours to avoid the sugar cravings. It has worked great for me.

CHOCOLATE: Allow one serving, twice a week. Note the amount eaten today:	
CARBONATED BEVERAGES: Drink one "1/2 can," 3 times a week. Write 0 to indicate that you did not consume any today, or 1,2 or 3 for the first, second or third "1/2 can" this week.	
COFFEE: Drink only one "1/2 cup" 3 times a week. Write 0 to indicate if you did not have any cups, or 1,2 or 3 for the first, second or third cup of the week.	
ALCOHOL: In the space indicate your first and second drink of this 30 day period. Write in a 0 if you did not imbibe.	
REFINED SUGARS: Limit sugar consumption to once every other day and white bread to 2 servings a day. Enter number of servings consumed:	
WATER: Drink 8 glasses of water. Amount consumed today:	
EXERCISE: Walk briskly for 30 minutes without stopping. Check here when finished.	
STRETCHING: Do exercise Plan #2. Check here when finished.	
SLEEP: Utilize ideas from the chapter on "Natural Sleep Aids."	
SUPPLEMENTS: Check here after taking your supplements.	
Breakfast:	
Lunch:	
Dinner:	
ON A SCALE OF 1-10, with 1 indicating that you are free of symptoms, rate how you feel today:	
Today's High Temperature:	

Briefly Describe Today's Weather:

What I Accomplished Today:

DAY 63

Remember that you didn't get this sickness overnight. You've probably had some of many of the symptoms for a long time. It will take a while for your body to heal itself.

CHOCOLATE: Allow one serving, twice a week. Note the amount eaten today:	
CARBONATED BEVERAGES: Drink one "1/2 can," 3 times a week. Write 0 to indicate that you did not consume any today, or 1,2 or 3 for the first, second or third "1/2 can" this week.	
COFFEE: Drink only one "1/2 cup" 3 times a week. Write 0 to indicate if you did not have any cups, or 1,2 or 3 for the first, second or third cup of the week.	
ALCOHOL: In the space indicate your first and second drink of this 30 day period. Write in a 0 if you did not imbibe.	
REFINED SUGARS: Limit sugar consumption to once every other day and white bread to 2 servings a day. Enter number of servings consumed:	
WATER: Drink 8 glasses of water. Amount consumed today:	
EXERCISE: Walk briskly for 30 minutes without stopping. Check here when finished.	
STRETCHING: Do exercise Plan #3. Check here when finished.	
SLEEP: Utilize ideas from the chapter on "Natural Sleep Aids."	
SUPPLEMENTS: Check here after taking your supplements.	
Breakfast:	
Lunch:	
Dinner:	
ON A SCALE OF 1-10, with 1 indicating that you are free of symptoms, rate how you feel today:	
Today's High Temperature:	

Briefly Describe Today's Weather:

What I Accomplished Today:

DAY 64

Supplements were very important for Kelly and my recovery. Be sure to use quality supplements. I have very poor results when using the generic brands.

CHOCOLATE: Allow one serving, twice a week. Note the amount eaten today:	
CARBONATED BEVERAGES: Drink one "1/2 can," 3 times a week. Write 0 to indicate that you did not consume any today, or 1,2 or 3 for the first, second or third "1/2 can" this week.	
COFFEE: Drink only one "1/2 cup" 3 times a week. Write 0 to indicate if you did not have any cups, or 1,2 or 3 for the first, second or third cup of the week.	
ALCOHOL: In the space indicate your first and second drink of this 30 day period. Write in a 0 if you did not imbibe.	
REFINED SUGARS: Limit sugar consumption to once every other day and white bread to 2 servings a day. Enter number of servings consumed:	
WATER: Drink 8 glasses of water. Amount consumed today:	
EXERCISE: Walk briskly for 30 minutes without stopping. Check here when finished.	
STRETCHING: Do exercise Plan #1. Check here when finished.	
SLEEP: Utilize ideas from the chapter on "Natural Sleep Aids."	
SUPPLEMENTS: Check here after taking your supplements.	
Breakfast:	
Lunch:	
Dinner:	
ON A SCALE OF 1-10, with 1 indicating that you are free of symptoms, rate how you feel today:	
Today's High Temperature:	

Briefly Describe Today's Weather:

What I Accomplished Today:

DAY 65

Mineral supplements have been an important addition to my diet. I always take my mineral supplements with food to avoid an upset stomach.

CHOCOLATE: Allow one serving, twice a week. Note the amount eaten today:	
CARBONATED BEVERAGES: Drink one "1/2 can," 3 times a week. Write 0 to indicate that you did not consume any today, or 1,2 or 3 for the first, second or third "1/2 can" this week.	
COFFEE: Drink only one "1/2 cup" 3 times a week. Write 0 to indicate if you did not have any cups, or 1,2 or 3 for the first, second or third cup of the week.	
ALCOHOL: In the space indicate your first and second drink of this 30 day period. Write in a 0 if you did not imbibe.	
REFINED SUGARS: Limit sugar consumption to once every other day and white bread to 2 servings a day. Enter number of servings consumed:	
WATER: Drink 8 glasses of water. Amount consumed today:	
EXERCISE: Walk briskly for 30 minutes without stopping. Check here when finished.	
STRETCHING: Do exercise Plan #2. Check here when finished.	
SLEEP: Utilize ideas from the chapter on "Natural Sleep Aids."	
SUPPLEMENTS: Check here after taking your supplements.	
Breakfast:	
Lunch:	
Dinner:	
ON A SCALE OF 1-10, with 1 indicating that you are free of symptoms, rate how you feel today:	
Today's High Temperature:	

Briefly Describe Today's Weather:

What I Accomplished Today:

DAY 66

Parsley is very nutritious and makes a pretty plant for flower beds. One to two handfuls of fresh parsley eaten daily can provide a hearty dose of many vitamins and minerals, including calcium.

CHOCOLATE: Allow one serving, twice a week. Note the amount eaten today:	
CARBONATED BEVERAGES: Drink one "1/2 can," 3 times a week. Write 0 to indicate that you did not consume any today, or 1,2 or 3 for the first, second or third "1/2 can" this week.	
COFFEE: Drink only one "1/2 cup" 3 times a week. Write 0 to indicate if you did not have any cups, or 1,2 or 3 for the first, second or third cup of the week.	
ALCOHOL: In the space indicate your first and second drink of this 30 day period. Write in a 0 if you did not imbibe.	
REFINED SUGARS: Limit sugar consumption to once every other day and white bread to 2 servings a day. Enter number of servings consumed:	
WATER: Drink 8 glasses of water. Amount consumed today:	
EXERCISE: Walk briskly for 30 minutes without stopping. Check here when finished.	
STRETCHING: Do exercise Plan #3. Check here when finished.	
SLEEP: Utilize ideas from the chapter on "Natural Sleep Aids."	
SUPPLEMENTS: Check here after taking your supplements.	
Breakfast:	
Lunch:	
Dinner:	
ON A SCALE OF 1-10, with 1 indicating that you are free of symptoms, rate how you feel today:	
Today's High Temperature:	

Briefly Describe Today's Weather:

What I Accomplished Today:

DAY 67

Parsley has been used as a diuretic and liver tonic to break up kidney stones and to soothe coughs. Parsley also makes a good addition to diets for people who have problems with anemia.

CHOCOLATE: Allow one serving, twice a week. Note the amount eaten today:	
CARBONATED BEVERAGES: Drink one "1/2 can," 3 times a week. Write 0 to indicate that you did not consume any today, or 1,2 or 3 for the first, second or third "1/2 can" this week.	
COFFEE: Drink only one "1/2 cup" 3 times a week. Write 0 to indicate if you did not have any cups, or 1,2 or 3 for the first, second or third cup of the week.	
ALCOHOL: In the space indicate your first and second drink of this 30 day period. Write in a 0 if you did not imbibe.	
REFINED SUGARS: Limit sugar consumption to once every other day and white bread to 2 servings a day. Enter number of servings consumed:	
WATER: Drink 8 glasses of water. Amount consumed today:	
EXERCISE: Walk briskly for 30 minutes without stopping. Check here when finished.	
STRETCHING: Do exercise Plan #1. Check here when finished.	
SLEEP: Utilize ideas from the chapter on "Natural Sleep Aids."	
SUPPLEMENTS: Check here after taking your supplements.	
Breakfast:	
Lunch:	
Dinner:	
ON A SCALE OF 1-10, with 1 indicating that you are free of symptoms, rate how you feel today:	
Today's High Temperature:	

Briefly Describe Today's Weather:

What I Accomplished Today:

DAY 68

Keep in mind that too much fresh parsley can irritate the kidneys. Eat no more than two handfuls of parsley a day.

CHOCOLATE: Allow one serving, twice a week. Note the amount eaten today:	
CARBONATED BEVERAGES: Drink one "1/2 can," 3 times a week. Write 0 to indicate that you did not consume any today, or 1,2 or 3 for the first, second or third "1/2 can" this week.	
COFFEE: Drink only one "1/2 cup" 3 times a week. Write 0 to indicate if you did not have any cups, or 1,2 or 3 for the first, second or third cup of the week.	
ALCOHOL: In the space indicate your first and second drink of this 30 day period. Write in a 0 if you did not imbibe.	
REFINED SUGARS: Limit sugar consumption to once every other day and white bread to 2 servings a day. Enter number of servings consumed:	
WATER: Drink 8 glasses of water. Amount consumed today:	
EXERCISE: Walk briskly for 30 minutes without stopping. Check here when finished.	
STRETCHING: Do exercise Plan #2. Check here when finished.	
SLEEP: Utilize ideas from the chapter on "Natural Sleep Aids."	
SUPPLEMENTS: Check here after taking your supplements.	
Breakfast:	
Lunch:	
Dinner:	
ON A SCALE OF 1-10, with 1 indicating that you are free of symptoms, rate how you feel today:	
Today's High Temperature:	

Briefly Describe Today's Weather:

What I Accomplished Today:

DAY 69

It is important to eat as many fresh fruits and vegetables as possible.

CHOCOLATE: Allow one serving, twice a week. Note the amount eaten today:	
CARBONATED BEVERAGES: Drink one "1/2 can," 3 times a week. Write 0 to indicate that you did not consume any today, or 1,2 or 3 for the first, second or third "1/2 can" this week.	
COFFEE: Drink only one "1/2 cup" 3 times a week. Write 0 to indicate if you did not have any cups, or 1,2 or 3 for the first, second or third cup of the week.	
ALCOHOL: In the space indicate your first and second drink of this 30 day period. Write in a 0 if you did not imbibe.	
REFINED SUGARS: Limit sugar consumption to once every other day and white bread to 2 servings a day. Enter number of servings consumed:	
WATER: Drink 8 glasses of water. Amount consumed today:	
EXERCISE: Walk briskly for 30 minutes without stopping. Check here when finished.	
STRETCHING: Do exercise Plan #3. Check here when finished.	
SLEEP: Utilize ideas from the chapter on "Natural Sleep Aids."	
SUPPLEMENTS: Check here after taking your supplements.	
Breakfast:	
Lunch:	
Dinner:	
ON A SCALE OF 1-10, with 1 indicating that you are free of symptoms, rate how you feel today:	
Today's High Temperature:	

Briefly Describe Today's Weather:

What I Accomplished Today:

DAY 70

Since our bodies many times don't metabolize foods as efficiently as they should or could, the amount of nutrients we receive from the food we eat could be much less than a person without FMS. When we eat foods that have been cooked, many of the nutrients are lost due to the cooking process. Since our bodies may not utilize the nutrients in our foods as well as healthy bodies, we are probably getting even fewer nutrients from cooked foods than a healthy person would get.

CHOCOLATE: Allow one serving, twice a week. Note the amount eaten today:	
CARBONATED BEVERAGES: Drink one "1/2 can," 3 times a week. Write 0 to indicate that you did not consume any today, or 1,2 or 3 for the first, second or third "1/2 can" this week.	
COFFEE: Drink only one "1/2 cup" 3 times a week. Write 0 to indicate if you did not have any cups, or 1,2 or 3 for the first, second or third cup of the week.	
ALCOHOL: In the space indicate your first and second drink of this 30 day period. Write in a 0 if you did not imbibe.	
REFINED SUGARS: Limit sugar consumption to once every other day and white bread to 2 servings a day. Enter number of servings consumed:	
WATER: Drink 8 glasses of water. Amount consumed today:	
EXERCISE: Walk briskly for 30 minutes without stopping. Check here when finished.	
STRETCHING: Do exercise Plan #1. Check here when finished.	
SLEEP: Utilize ideas from the chapter on "Natural Sleep Aids."	
SUPPLEMENTS: Check here after taking your supplements.	
Breakfast:	
Lunch:	
Dinner:	
ON A SCALE OF 1-10, with 1 indicating that you are free of symptoms, rate how you feel today:	
Today's High Temperature:	

Briefly Describe Today's Weather:

What I Accomplished Today:

DAY 71

Once I started eating more fresh fruits and vegetables, I noticed an increase in energy. Regardless of the time of year, start trying new "summer" recipes, which usually include more fresh fruits and vegetables.

CHOCOLATE: Allow one serving, twice a week. Note the amount eaten today:	
CARBONATED BEVERAGES: Drink one "1/2 can," 3 times a week. Write 0 to indicate that you did not consume any today, or 1,2 or 3 for the first, second or third "1/2 can" this week.	
COFFEE: Drink only one "1/2 cup" 3 times a week. Write 0 to indicate if you did not have any cups, or 1,2 or 3 for the first, second or third cup of the week.	
ALCOHOL: In the space indicate your first and second drink of this 30 day period. Write in a 0 if you did not imbibe.	
REFINED SUGARS: Limit sugar consumption to once every other day and white bread to 2 servings a day. Enter number of servings consumed:	
WATER: Drink 8 glasses of water. Amount consumed today:	
EXERCISE: Walk briskly for 30 minutes without stopping. Check here when finished.	
STRETCHING: Do exercise Plan #2. Check here when finished.	
SLEEP: Utilize ideas from the chapter on "Natural Sleep Aids."	
SUPPLEMENTS: Check here after taking your supplements.	
Breakfast:	
Lunch:	
Dinner:	
ON A SCALE OF 1-10, with 1 indicating that you are free of symptoms, rate how you feel today:	
Today's High Temperature:	

Briefly Describe Today's Weather:

What I Accomplished Today:

DAY 72

To make a fast, easy, accessible meal, try mixing broccoli, cauliflower, carrots, peppers and celery in a food processor. Keep the salad in the freezer or refrigerator until you want to use it. Put you favorite dressing on it for a flavorful, healthy meal. These vegetables are also good on top of lettuce or in soup.

CHOCOLATE: Allow one serving, twice a week. Note the amount eaten today:	
CARBONATED BEVERAGES: Drink one "1/2 can," 3 times a week. Write 0 to indicate that you did not consume any today, or 1,2 or 3 for the first, second or third "1/2 can" this week.	
COFFEE: Drink only one "1/2 cup" 3 times a week. Write 0 to indicate if you did not have any cups, or 1,2 or 3 for the first, second or third cup of the week.	
ALCOHOL: In the space indicate your first and second drink of this 30 day period. Write in a 0 if you did not imbibe.	
REFINED SUGARS: Limit sugar consumption to once every other day and white bread to 2 servings a day. Enter number of servings consumed:	
WATER: Drink 8 glasses of water. Amount consumed today:	
EXERCISE: Walk briskly for 30 minutes without stopping. Check here when finished.	
STRETCHING: Do exercise Plan #3. Check here when finished.	
SLEEP: Utilize ideas from the chapter on "Natural Sleep Aids."	
SUPPLEMENTS: Check here after taking your supplements.	
Breakfast:	
Lunch:	
Dinner:	
ON A SCALE OF 1-10, with 1 indicating that you are free of symptoms, rate how you feel today:	
Today's High Temperature:	

Briefly Describe Today's Weather:

What I Accomplished Today:

DAY 73

Garlic is a wonderful herb to add to your diet and garden. Garlic has an old reputation of helping to lower blood pressure. I stated earlier in this book, be careful to not over do it.

CHOCOLATE: Allow one serving, twice a week. Note the amount eaten today:	
CARBONATED BEVERAGES: Drink one "1/2 can," 3 times a week. Write 0 to indicate that you did not consume any today, or 1,2 or 3 for the first, second or third "1/2 can" this week.	
COFFEE: Drink only one "1/2 cup" 3 times a week. Write 0 to indicate if you did not have any cups, or 1,2 or 3 for the first, second or third cup of the week.	
ALCOHOL: In the space indicate your first and second drink of this 30 day period. Write in a 0 if you did not imbibe.	
REFINED SUGARS: Limit sugar consumption to once every other day and white bread to 2 servings a day. Enter number of servings consumed:	
WATER: Drink 8 glasses of water. Amount consumed today:	
EXERCISE: Walk briskly for 30 minutes without stopping. Check here when finished.	
STRETCHING: Do exercise Plan #3. Check here when finished.	
SLEEP: Utilize ideas from the chapter on "Natural Sleep Aids."	
SUPPLEMENTS: Check here after taking your supplements.	
Breakfast:	
Lunch:	
Dinner:	
ON A SCALE OF 1-10, with 1 indicating that you are free of symptoms, rate how you feel today:	
Today's High Temperature:	

Briefly Describe Today's Weather:

What I Accomplished Today:

DAY 74

If your symptoms of pain are caused from candida (yeast) overgrowth, there are a number of natural remedies that may be of help. Garlic is one of the herbs that help control candida.

CHOCOLATE: Allow one serving, twice a week. Note the amount eaten today:	
CARBONATED BEVERAGES: Drink one "1/2 can," 3 times a week. Write 0 to indicate that you did not consume any today, or 1,2 or 3 for the first, second or third "1/2 can" this week.	
COFFEE: Drink only one "1/2 cup" 3 times a week. Write 0 to indicate if you did not have any cups, or 1,2 or 3 for the first, second or third cup of the week.	
ALCOHOL: In the space indicate your first and second drink of this 30 day period. Write in a 0 if you did not imbibe.	
REFINED SUGARS: Limit sugar consumption to once every other day and white bread to 2 servings a day. Enter number of servings consumed:	
WATER: Drink 8 glasses of water. Amount consumed today:	
EXERCISE: Walk briskly for 30 minutes without stopping. Check here when finished.	
STRETCHING: Do exercise Plan #1. Check here when finished.	
SLEEP: Utilize ideas from the chapter on "Natural Sleep Aids."	
SUPPLEMENTS: Check here after taking your supplements.	
Breakfast:	
Lunch:	
Dinner:	
ON A SCALE OF 1-10, with 1 indicating that you are free of symptoms, rate how you feel today:	
Today's High Temperature:	

Briefly Describe Today's Weather:

What I Accomplished Today:

DAY 75

Garlic planted around fruit and nut trees will help keep moles away. Planted around rose bushes, garlic will help repel aphids.

CHOCOLATE: Allow one serving, twice a week. Note the amount eaten today:	
CARBONATED BEVERAGES: Drink one "1/2 can," 3 times a week. Write 0 to indicate that you did not consume any today, or 1,2 or 3 for the first, second or third "1/2 can" this week.	
COFFEE: Drink only one "1/2 cup" 3 times a week. Write 0 to indicate if you did not have any cups, or 1,2 or 3 for the first, second or third cup of the week.	
ALCOHOL: In the space indicate your first and second drink of this 30 day period. Write in a 0 if you did not imbibe.	
REFINED SUGARS: Limit sugar consumption to once every other day and white bread to 2 servings a day. Enter number of servings consumed:	
WATER: Drink 8 glasses of water. Amount consumed today:	
EXERCISE: Walk briskly for 30 minutes without stopping. Check here when finished.	
STRETCHING: Do exercise Plan #2. Check here when finished.	
SLEEP: Utilize ideas from the chapter on "Natural Sleep Aids."	
SUPPLEMENTS: Check here after taking your supplements.	
Breakfast:	
Lunch:	
Dinner:	
ON A SCALE OF 1-10, with 1 indicating that you are free of symptoms, rate how you feel today:	
Today's High Temperature:	

Briefly Describe Today's Weather:

What I Accomplished Today:

DAY 76

A couple of years ago, I noticed some ants that had made their way into our home via a small crack in the window sill. Garlic worked wonders in keeping them at bay. I pour some garlic tea in my window sills to keep black ants away. You may not want to pour the tea in your window sills if you don't have an area for the tea to drain out of the sills!

CHOCOLATE: Allow one serving, twice a week. Note the amount eaten today:	
CARBONATED BEVERAGES: Drink one "1/2 can," 3 times a week. Write 0 to indicate that you did not consume any today, or 1,2 or 3 for the first, second or third "1/2 can" this week.	
COFFEE: Drink only one "1/2 cup" 3 times a week. Write 0 to indicate if you did not have any cups, or 1,2 or 3 for the first, second or third cup of the week.	
ALCOHOL: In the space indicate your first and second drink of this 30 day period. Write in a 0 if you did not imbibe.	
REFINED SUGARS: Limit sugar consumption to once every other day and white bread to 2 servings a day. Enter number of servings consumed:	
WATER: Drink 8 glasses of water. Amount consumed today:	
EXERCISE: Walk briskly for 30 minutes without stopping. Check here when finished.	
STRETCHING: Do exercise Plan #3. Check here when finished.	
SLEEP: Utilize ideas from the chapter on "Natural Sleep Aids."	
SUPPLEMENTS: Check here after taking your supplements.	
Breakfast:	
Lunch:	
Dinner:	
ON A SCALE OF 1-10, with 1 indicating that you are free of symptoms, rate how you feel today:	
Today's High Temperature:	

Briefly Describe Today's Weather:

What I Accomplished Today:

DAY 77

A wonderful way to use garlic to enhance spaghetti, noodles, etc., is to sauté fresh garlic and parsley in two tablespoons of olive oil. Then toss the spaghetti in the oil mixture.

CHOCOLATE: Allow one serving, twice a week. Note the amount eaten today:	
CARBONATED BEVERAGES: Drink one "1/2 can," 3 times a week. Write 0 to indicate that you did not consume any today, or 1,2 or 3 for the first, second or third "1/2 can" this week.	
COFFEE: Drink only one "1/2 cup" 3 times a week. Write 0 to indicate if you did not have any cups, or 1,2 or 3 for the first, second or third cup of the week.	
ALCOHOL: In the space indicate your first and second drink of this 30 day period. Write in a 0 if you did not imbibe.	
REFINED SUGARS: Limit sugar consumption to once every other day and white bread to 2 servings a day. Enter number of servings consumed:	
WATER: Drink 8 glasses of water. Amount consumed today:	
EXERCISE: Walk briskly for 30 minutes without stopping. Check here when finished.	
STRETCHING: Do exercise Plan #1. Check here when finished.	
SLEEP: Utilize ideas from the chapter on "Natural Sleep Aids."	
SUPPLEMENTS: Check here after taking your supplements.	
Breakfast:	
Lunch:	
Dinner:	
ON A SCALE OF 1-10, with 1 indicating that you are free of symptoms, rate how you feel today:	
Today's High Temperature:	

Briefly Describe Today's Weather:

What I Accomplished Today:

DAY 78

You're doing well. If you've slipped a little, give yourself a break. You can always start fresh again tomorrow.

CHOCOLATE: Allow one serving, twice a week. Note the amount eaten today:	
CARBONATED BEVERAGES: Drink one "1/2 can," 3 times a week. Write 0 to indicate that you did not consume any today, or 1,2 or 3 for the first, second or third "1/2 can" this week.	
COFFEE: Drink only one "1/2 cup" 3 times a week. Write 0 to indicate if you did not have any cups, or 1,2 or 3 for the first, second or third cup of the week.	
ALCOHOL: In the space indicate your first and second drink of this 30 day period. Write in a 0 if you did not imbibe.	
REFINED SUGARS: Limit sugar consumption to once every other day and white bread to 2 servings a day. Enter number of servings consumed:	
WATER: Drink 8 glasses of water. Amount consumed today:	
EXERCISE: Walk briskly for 30 minutes without stopping. Check here when finished.	
STRETCHING: Do exercise Plan #2. Check here when finished.	
SLEEP: Utilize ideas from the chapter on "Natural Sleep Aids."	
SUPPLEMENTS: Check here after taking your supplements.	
Breakfast:	
Lunch:	
Dinner:	
ON A SCALE OF 1-10, with 1 indicating that you are free of symptoms, rate how you feel today:	
Today's High Temperature:	

Briefly Describe Today's Weather:

What I Accomplished Today:

DAY 79

Remember that the goal is to eliminate completely from our diets the following: chocolate, carbonated beverages, coffee, and alcohol. Many times people tell me that if they must eat so healthy, they just as well not be alive because life isn't worth living if a person has to give up all the "good" things in life to feel well. Once I changed my attitude and focus, a noticeable physical healing began to take place. I would rather enjoy the hours of fun and be able to do everything else I had wanted to do for so long, but didn't fell well enough to do, than worry about 20 minutes of food three times a day. What do you think?

CHOCOLATE: Allow one serving, twice a week. Note the amount eaten today:	
CARBONATED BEVERAGES: Drink one "1/2 can," 3 times a week. Write 0 to indicate that you did not consume any today, or 1,2 or 3 for the first, second or third "1/2 can" this week.	
COFFEE: Drink only one "1/2 cup" 3 times a week. Write 0 to indicate if you did not have any cups, or 1,2 or 3 for the first, second or third cup of the week.	
ALCOHOL: In the space indicate your first and second drink of this 30 day period. Write in a 0 if you did not imbibe.	
REFINED SUGARS: Limit sugar consumption to once every other day and white bread to 2 servings a day. Enter number of servings consumed:	
WATER: Drink 8 glasses of water. Amount consumed today:	
EXERCISE: Walk briskly for 30 minutes without stopping. Check here when finished.	
STRETCHING: Do exercise Plan #3. Check here when finished.	
SLEEP: Utilize ideas from the chapter on "Natural Sleep Aids."	
SUPPLEMENTS: Check here after taking your supplements.	
Breakfast:	
Lunch:	
Dinner:	
ON A SCALE OF 1-10, with 1 indicating that you are free of symptoms, rate how you feel today:	
Today's High Temperature:	

Briefly Describe Today's Weather:

What I Accomplished Today:

DAY 80

I am very careful to watch for preservatives, such as MSG in foods. Many canned soups contain MSG. Be sure to check labels of soup products to be sure there is no MSG present.

CHOCOLATE: Allow one serving, twice a week. Note the amount eaten today:	
CARBONATED BEVERAGES: Drink one "1/2 can," 3 times a week. Write 0 to indicate that you did not consume any today, or 1,2 or 3 for the first, second or third "1/2 can" this week.	
COFFEE: Drink only one "1/2 cup" 3 times a week. Write 0 to indicate if you did not have any cups, or 1,2 or 3 for the first, second or third cup of the week.	
ALCOHOL: In the space indicate your first and second drink of this 30 day period. Write in a 0 if you did not imbibe.	
REFINED SUGARS: Limit sugar consumption to once every other day and white bread to 2 servings a day. Enter number of servings consumed:	
WATER: Drink 8 glasses of water. Amount consumed today:	
EXERCISE: Walk briskly for 30 minutes without stopping. Check here when finished.	
STRETCHING: Do exercise Plan #1. Check here when finished.	
SLEEP: Utilize ideas from the chapter on "Natural Sleep Aids."	
SUPPLEMENTS: Check here after taking your supplements.	
Breakfast:	
Lunch:	
Dinner:	
ON A SCALE OF 1-10, with 1 indicating that you are free of symptoms, rate how you feel today:	
Today's High Temperature:	

Briefly Describe Today's Weather:

What I Accomplished Today:

DAY 81

Recently we took a trip to Branson, Missouri, and while there we went into a store in a mall. In this store were about 10 people handing out samples of snack foods to customers as they walked in the door. Within 25 minutes after walking into the door of that store I had a horrible headache. Aspirin didn't faze this headache, so I had to go back to the motel and do a massage treatment on my legs to get rid of the headache.

CHOCOLATE: Allow one serving, twice a week. Note the amount eaten today:	
CARBONATED BEVERAGES: Drink one "1/2 can," 3 times a week. Write 0 to indicate that you did not consume any today, or 1,2 or 3 for the first, second or third "1/2 can" this week.	
COFFEE: Drink only one "1/2 cup" 3 times a week. Write 0 to indicate if you did not have any cups, or 1,2 or 3 for the first, second or third cup of the week.	
ALCOHOL: In the space indicate your first and second drink of this 30 day period. Write in a 0 if you did not imbibe.	
REFINED SUGARS: Limit sugar consumption to once every other day and white bread to 2 servings a day. Enter number of servings consumed:	
WATER: Drink 8 glasses of water. Amount consumed today:	
EXERCISE: Walk briskly for 30 minutes without stopping. Check here when finished.	
STRETCHING: Do exercise Plan #2. Check here when finished.	
SLEEP: Utilize ideas from the chapter on "Natural Sleep Aids."	
SUPPLEMENTS: Check here after taking your supplements.	
Breakfast:	
Lunch:	
Dinner:	
ON A SCALE OF 1-10, with 1 indicating that you are free of symptoms, rate how you feel today:	
Today's High Temperature:	

Briefly Describe Today's Weather:

What I Accomplished Today:

DAY 82

Once again I would like to accentuate the necessity of minerals in my diet. As I said earlier, there are some minerals that people with FMS seem to be deficient in. Those are magnesium, manganese, folic acid, the B vitamins, zinc, calcium and vitamin C.

CHOCOLATE: Allow one serving, twice a week. Note the amount eaten today:	
CARBONATED BEVERAGES: Drink one "1/2 can," 3 times a week. Write 0 to indicate that you did not consume any today, or 1,2 or 3 for the first, second or third "1/2 can" this week.	
COFFEE: Drink only one "1/2 cup" 3 times a week. Write 0 to indicate if you did not have any cups, or 1,2 or 3 for the first, second or third cup of the week.	
ALCOHOL: In the space indicate your first and second drink of this 30 day period. Write in a 0 if you did not imbibe.	
REFINED SUGARS: Limit sugar consumption to once every other day and white bread to 2 servings a day. Enter number of servings consumed:	
WATER: Drink 8 glasses of water. Amount consumed today:	
EXERCISE: Walk briskly for 30 minutes without stopping. Check here when finished.	
STRETCHING: Do exercise Plan #3. Check here when finished.	
SLEEP: Utilize ideas from the chapter on "Natural Sleep Aids."	
SUPPLEMENTS: Check here after taking your supplements.	
Breakfast:	
Lunch:	
Dinner:	
ON A SCALE OF 1-10, with 1 indicating that you are free of symptoms, rate how you feel today:	
Today's High Temperature:	

Briefly Describe Today's Weather:

What I Accomplished Today:

DAY 83

In the early days of my healing process, I found it to be very difficult to limit sweets. I found it was helpful to allow a tiny serving one time a week, usually on the weekend. I looked forward to my "sweet treat," although I could feel the ill effects it had on my body almost immediately.

CHOCOLATE: Allow one serving, twice a week. Note the amount eaten today:	
CARBONATED BEVERAGES: Drink one "1/2 can," 3 times a week. Write 0 to indicate that you did not consume any today, or 1,2 or 3 for the first, second or third "1/2 can" this week.	
COFFEE: Drink only one "1/2 cup" 3 times a week. Write 0 to indicate if you did not have any cups, or 1,2 or 3 for the first, second or third cup of the week.	
ALCOHOL: In the space indicate your first and second drink of this 30 day period. Write in a 0 if you did not imbibe.	
REFINED SUGARS: Limit sugar consumption to once every other day and white bread to 2 servings a day. Enter number of servings consumed:	
WATER: Drink 8 glasses of water. Amount consumed today:	
EXERCISE: Walk briskly for 30 minutes without stopping. Check here when finished.	
STRETCHING: Do exercise Plan #1. Check here when finished.	
SLEEP: Utilize ideas from the chapter on "Natural Sleep Aids."	
SUPPLEMENTS: Check here after taking your supplements.	
Breakfast:	
Lunch:	
Dinner:	
ON A SCALE OF 1-10, with 1 indicating that you are free of symptoms, rate how you feel today:	
Today's High Temperature:	

Briefly Describe Today's Weather:

What I Accomplished Today:

DAY 84

Sugar added to our diets can make them a complete disaster. Refined sugar actually helps to break down our immune system, which could make us more susceptible to immune problems.

CHOCOLATE: Allow one serving, twice a week. Note the amount eaten today:	
CARBONATED BEVERAGES: Drink one "1/2 can," 3 times a week. Write 0 to indicate that you did not consume any today, or 1,2 or 3 for the first, second or third "1/2 can" this week.	
COFFEE: Drink only one "1/2 cup" 3 times a week. Write 0 to indicate if you did not have any cups, or 1,2 or 3 for the first, second or third cup of the week.	
ALCOHOL: In the space indicate your first and second drink of this 30 day period. Write in a 0 if you did not imbibe.	
REFINED SUGARS: Limit sugar consumption to once every other day and white bread to 2 servings a day. Enter number of servings consumed:	
WATER: Drink 8 glasses of water. Amount consumed today:	
EXERCISE: Walk briskly for 30 minutes without stopping. Check here when finished.	
STRETCHING: Do exercise Plan #2. Check here when finished.	
SLEEP: Utilize ideas from the chapter on "Natural Sleep Aids."	
SUPPLEMENTS: Check here after taking your supplements.	
Breakfast:	
Lunch:	
Dinner:	
ON A SCALE OF 1-10, with 1 indicating that you are free of symptoms, rate how you feel today:	
Today's High Temperature:	

Briefly Describe Today's Weather:

What I Accomplished Today:

DAY 85

The various pieces of information contained in this book are "tools" to help you feel good again. You can feel good again, but it's up to you to make the necessary changes. And actually, since you made it to Day 85, it is obvious that you are serious about achieving your goals!

CHOCOLATE: Allow one serving, twice a week. Note the amount eaten today:	
CARBONATED BEVERAGES: Drink one "1/2 can," 3 times a week. Write 0 to indicate that you did not consume any today, or 1,2 or 3 for the first, second or third "1/2 can" this week.	
COFFEE: Drink only one "1/2 cup" 3 times a week. Write 0 to indicate if you did not have any cups, or 1,2 or 3 for the first, second or third cup of the week.	
ALCOHOL: In the space indicate your first and second drink of this 30 day period. Write in a 0 if you did not imbibe.	
REFINED SUGARS: Limit sugar consumption to once every other day and white bread to 2 servings a day. Enter number of servings consumed:	
WATER: Drink 8 glasses of water. Amount consumed today:	
EXERCISE: Walk briskly for 30 minutes without stopping. Check here when finished.	
STRETCHING: Do exercise Plan #3. Check here when finished.	
SLEEP: Utilize ideas from the chapter on "Natural Sleep Aids."	
SUPPLEMENTS: Check here after taking your supplements.	
Breakfast:	
Lunch:	
Dinner:	
ON A SCALE OF 1-10, with 1 indicating that you are free of symptoms, rate how you feel today:	
Today's High Temperature:	

Briefly Describe Today's Weather:

What I Accomplished Today:

DAY 86

Part of my maintenance for keeping well has included regular chiropractic adjustments. It has been interesting to feel the differences in my body from when I felt bad compared to now. The adjustments I now need are generally due to back strain from gardening.

CHOCOLATE: Allow one serving, twice a week. Note the amount eaten today:	
CARBONATED BEVERAGES: Drink one "1/2 can," 3 times a week. Write 0 to indicate that you did not consume any today, or 1,2 or 3 for the first, second or third "1/2 can" this week.	
COFFEE: Drink only one "1/2 cup" 3 times a week. Write 0 to indicate if you did not have any cups, or 1,2 or 3 for the first, second or third cup of the week.	
ALCOHOL: In the space indicate your first and second drink of this 30 day period. Write in a 0 if you did not imbibe.	
REFINED SUGARS: Limit sugar consumption to once every other day and white bread to 2 servings a day. Enter number of servings consumed:	
WATER: Drink 8 glasses of water. Amount consumed today:	
EXERCISE: Walk briskly for 30 minutes without stopping. Check here when finished.	
STRETCHING: Do exercise Plan #3. Check here when finished.	
SLEEP: Utilize ideas from the chapter on "Natural Sleep Aids."	
SUPPLEMENTS: Check here after taking your supplements.	
Breakfast:	
Lunch:	
Dinner:	
ON A SCALE OF 1-10, with 1 indicating that you are free of symptoms, rate how you feel today:	
Today's High Temperature:	

Briefly Describe Today's Weather:

What I Accomplished Today:

DAY 87

Focus solely on the positive aspects of your life today.

CHOCOLATE: Allow one serving, twice a week. Note the amount eaten today:	
CARBONATED BEVERAGES: Drink one "1/2 can," 3 times a week. Write 0 to indicate that you did not consume any today, or 1,2 or 3 for the first, second or third "1/2 can" this week.	
COFFEE: Drink only one "1/2 cup" 3 times a week. Write 0 to indicate if you did not have any cups, or 1,2 or 3 for the first, second or third cup of the week.	
ALCOHOL: In the space indicate your first and second drink of this 30 day period. Write in a 0 if you did not imbibe.	
REFINED SUGARS: Limit sugar consumption to once every other day and white bread to 2 servings a day. Enter number of servings consumed:	
WATER: Drink 8 glasses of water. Amount consumed today:	
EXERCISE: Walk briskly for 30 minutes without stopping. Check here when finished.	
STRETCHING: Do exercise Plan #1. Check here when finished.	
SLEEP: Utilize ideas from the chapter on "Natural Sleep Aids."	
SUPPLEMENTS: Check here after taking your supplements.	
Breakfast:	
Lunch:	
Dinner:	
ON A SCALE OF 1-10, with 1 indicating that you are free of symptoms, rate how you feel today:	
Today's High Temperature:	

Briefly Describe Today's Weather:

What I Accomplished Today:

DAY 88

It is still important for me to take about 20 minutes every day to sit or lie in a comfortable place and just be still. I try not to think of anything, just be.

CHOCOLATE: Allow one serving, twice a week. Note the amount eaten today:	
CARBONATED BEVERAGES: Drink one "1/2 can," 3 times a week. Write 0 to indicate that you did not consume any today, or 1,2 or 3 for the first, second or third "1/2 can" this week.	
COFFEE: Drink only one "1/2 cup" 3 times a week. Write 0 to indicate if you did not have any cups, or 1,2 or 3 for the first, second or third cup of the week.	
ALCOHOL: In the space indicate your first and second drink of this 30 day period. Write in a 0 if you did not imbibe.	
REFINED SUGARS: Limit sugar consumption to once every other day and white bread to 2 servings a day. Enter number of servings consumed:	
WATER: Drink 8 glasses of water. Amount consumed today:	
EXERCISE: Walk briskly for 30 minutes without stopping. Check here when finished.	
STRETCHING: Do exercise Plan #2. Check here when finished.	
SLEEP: Utilize ideas from the chapter on "Natural Sleep Aids."	
SUPPLEMENTS: Check here after taking your supplements.	
Breakfast:	
Lunch:	
Dinner:	
ON A SCALE OF 1-10, with 1 indicating that you are free of symptoms, rate how you feel today:	
Today's High Temperature:	

Briefly Describe Today's Weather:

What I Accomplished Today:

DAY 89

Thinking positively is not so difficult to do once we accept the basic premise that there is a greater force that has built this beautiful home for us. I'm not thinking about a man made structure. Think about birds, plants and the earth, everything in life is as it should be, and we should be careful about how we impact it.

CHOCOLATE: Allow one serving, twice a week. Note the amount eaten today:	
CARBONATED BEVERAGES: Drink one "1/2 can," 3 times a week. Write 0 to indicate that you did not consume any today, or 1,2 or 3 for the first, second or third "1/2 can" this week.	
COFFEE: Drink only one "1/2 cup" 3 times a week. Write 0 to indicate if you did not have any cups, or 1,2 or 3 for the first, second or third cup of the week.	
ALCOHOL: In the space indicate your first and second drink of this 30 day period. Write in a 0 if you did not imbibe.	
REFINED SUGARS: Limit sugar consumption to once every other day and white bread to 2 servings a day. Enter number of servings consumed:	
WATER: Drink 8 glasses of water. Amount consumed today:	
EXERCISE: Walk briskly for 30 minutes without stopping. Check here when finished.	
STRETCHING: Do exercise Plan #3. Check here when finished.	
SLEEP: Utilize ideas from the chapter on "Natural Sleep Aids."	
SUPPLEMENTS: Check here after taking your supplements.	
Breakfast:	
Lunch:	
Dinner:	
ON A SCALE OF 1-10, with 1 indicating that you are free of symptoms, rate how you feel today:	
Today's High Temperature:	

Briefly Describe Today's Weather:

What I Accomplished Today:

DAY 90

You are great. You do not need this any more. You will set your own stringent standards and continue to work off of the foods which you should eliminate. You will also continue with all of your healthy sleeping and living habits. You have found the strength from within. Take a deep breath... and proceed with a big smile!

CHOCOLATE: Allow one serving,once a week for three weeks, then eliminate chocolate completely.	
CARBONATED BEVERAGES: Drink one "1/2 can," 3 times a week. Write 0 to indicate that you did not consume any today, or 1,2 or 3 for the first, second or third "1/2 can" this week.	
COFFEE: Drink only one "1/2 cup" 3 times a week. Write 0 to indicate if you did not have any cups, or 1,2 or 3 for the first, second or third cup of the week.	
ALCOHOL: In the space indicate your first and second drink of this 30 day period. Write in a 0 if you did not imbibe.	
REFINED SUGARS: Limit sugar consumption to once every other day and white bread to 2 servings a day. Enter number of servings consumed:	
WATER: Drink 8 glasses of water. Amount consumed today:	
EXERCISE: Walk briskly for 30 minutes without stopping. Check here when finished.	
STRETCHING: Do exercise Plan #1. Check here when finished.	
SLEEP: Utilize ideas from the chapter on "Natural Sleep Aids."	
SUPPLEMENTS: Check here after taking your supplements.	
Breakfast:	
Lunch:	
Dinner:	
ON A SCALE OF 1-10, with 1 indicating that you are free of symptoms, rate how you feel today:	
Today's High Temperature:	

Briefly Describe Today's Weather:

What I Accomplished Today:

HEALTH EVALUATION FORM

Indicate in the column next to the symptoms which of the following conditions apply to you in terms of frequency and/or intensity of symptoms using the numbers of 1-10: With 1 indicating the least and 10 indicating the greatest intensity or frequency.

Low Energy	____	Often Feel Tired	____	Headaches	____
Dry/itchy Skin	____	Dry or Itchy scalp	____	Rashes or Eczema	____
Achy Joints	____	Muscle Cramps	____	Muscle Twitches	____
Bruising	____	Menstrual Cramps	____	Moody/PMS	____
Poor Concentration	____	Water Retention	____	Bowel Gas	____
Numbing/Tingling	____	Skin Burning	____	Dry Eyes	____
Weak Fingernails	____	Dry/Brittle Hair	____	Weak Muscles	____
Joint Pain	____	Foot Pain	____	TMJ Pain	____

Indigestion/Acid Reflux	____	Constipation and/or Diarrhea	____
Frequently Take Pain Killers	____	Difficulty Handling Stress	____
High/Low Blood Pressure	____	Strong Desire for Sweets/Salts	____
Moods of Depression	____	Often feel Bloated	____
Cold Hands and Feet	____	Difficulty Falling Asleep	____
Shortness of Breath	____	Allergies and/or Hayfever	____
Poor Night Vision	____	Light Sleep/Aware of Surroundings	____

NOTE: Once you have completed this health evaluation, return to the previous health evaluations and compare the improvements. Make at least four extra copies of this evaluation for use once a month. Improvement will be gradual. By filling out the health evaluation monthly it will be easier to continue to see the progress your body is making during its healing process.

Peaceful Serenity

My favorite place is on the hilltop
Where I sit and pray.
To watch the peaceful sunrise
And contemplate my day.
And as the sun rises over the hill
The moon begins to fade;
The stones before me tell a life
Of those, within the grave.
This is my favorite place
To come and sit and rest.
The peace and serenity I find here
Is far above the best
The sun reminds me of wondrous life
Here upon the earth;
The moon is awesome in its glow
No price can show its worth.
The stones tell me the story
Of those who lived before.
And now know peace within a realm
Of some not so distant shore
Now as I stand to leave this place
The birds fly overhead
Singing songs of peace and joy
Ours on earth to spread.

Mary Moeller

Cold Turkey Technique

Some faire well with this fowl approach.

CHOCOLATE: Eliminate all chocolate.	
CARBONATED BEVERAGES: From now on, you will eliminate carbonated beverages from your diet.	
COFFEE: Beginning today, you will eliminate coffee from your diet.	
ALCOHOL: Beginning today you have eliminated alcohol from your diet.	
REFINED SUGARS: Limit sugars to 2 servings a week and breads and pastas to 3 servings per week.	
WATER: Drink 8 glasses of water every day.	
EXERCISE: Your goal is now to walk 40 minutes everyday. Walk briskly for 40 minutes without stopping	
STRETCHING: Stretch everyday. Alternate the stretching routines so that you complete all three twice a week.	
SLEEP: Use ideas from back of book.	
SUPPLEMENTS: Take supplements every day.	
Breakfast:	
Lunch:	
Dinner:	

Natural Sleep Aids

Being unable to get a good nights sleep is a complaint common to sufferers of fibromyalgia and chronic fatigue syndrome. Problems may range from difficulties in falling asleep and waking up numerous times during the night, to sleeping all night and waking in the morning feeling as though sleep has not happened at all. As the diet is changed, nutritional deficiencies met, and systemic yeast dies (for those who have a systemic yeast problem), sleep generally improves. The vast majority of those who diligently follow the protocol set forth in this book notice a great improvement in sleep within four weeks. As time continues and lifestyle changes are made, the number of hours of deep sleep increases and the number of waking periods during the night decreases. Organs continue to heal and falling back to sleep when one awakens becomes easier, until, finally, seven to eight hours of deep sleep is achieved. The time frame to notice improvements in sleep depends upon how diligently the program is followed.

In Chinese medicine, it is believed every two hours of the day and night a different organ restores itself. For every organ that is restoring itself, twelve hours later a complimentary organ restores itself. For each of these organs to be healthy and strong, the other must be healthy and strong. If one of the organs is weakened or not functioning properly, a person will probably wake up during the time of the night that one of the two organs would be restoring itself. Over and again, I have seen clients who have used my program begin to notice an improvement in their sleep within a short few weeks. Once sleeping a solid four to six hours, the Organ Restoring Times Chart can be followed.

ORGAN RESTORING TIMES CHART

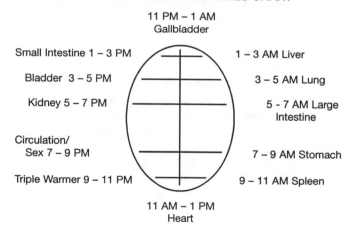

11 PM – 1 AM
Gallbladder

Small Intestine 1 – 3 PM

Bladder 3 – 5 PM

Kidney 5 – 7 PM

Circulation/
Sex 7 – 9 PM

Triple Warmer 9 – 11 PM

1 – 3 AM Liver

3 – 5 AM Lung

5 - 7 AM Large
Intestine

7 – 9 AM Stomach

9 – 11 AM Spleen

11 AM – 1 PM
Heart

I will illustrate how to use this chart by telling the story of my client, Rachael. When I began working with Rachael, she was waking up every hour or two. Within four weeks of following the lifestyle changes and nutritional program she was sleeping a solid four and one-half hours. She would generally fall asleep around ten o'clock at night and wake up around two thirty in the morning. In looking at the Organ Restoring Times Chart, we see that the organ that restores itself from one to three in the morning is the liver. Its complimentary organ is the small intestine. In testing to see which organ or organs were weakened by using a reflexology chart, the acupuncture meridian chart and the muscles that relate to those organs through Touch for Health, we confirmed that the liver was the organ that was waking Rachael at that time of the morning. A number of acupressure points, foods and herbs that are helpful in restoring the liver to health were suggested. When Rachael and I visited two weeks later, she was sleeping until four thirty in the morning. Once again, we followed the guidelines in determining organ weakness pertinent to that time, offered suggestions of acupressure points, herbs and foods helpful in restoring those organs, and within another three weeks Rachael was sleeping through the entire night, without medications!

Until the organs heal, there are a number of natural ways to help induce or deepen sleep. The following are common remedies which can be used to help improve your sleep:

Acupressure

Acupressure is one of the most effective self-administered treatments for sleep disturbances sufferers can use. Combined with dietary changes and nutritional supplementation, many find they fall asleep almost immediately once the body becomes accustomed to the use of acupressure. Although results may be immediate, it may take a number of months to change overall sleep patterns through the use of acupressure. For information on points to use for sleep, refer to the section on acupressure.

Acupuncture

Acupuncture can be a very effective tool for sleep disorders and in relieving pain. It has been my experience that not all acupuncturists are effective in treating fibromyalgia related symptoms. Before receiving a treatment from an acupuncturist, it is important to know a little about what to look for in an acupuncturist who would be more knowledgeable in treating fibromyalgia. Ask questions, such as, "How much training have you had?" before making an appointment. Many states require very few hours to receive an acupuncturist license. Ask if the acupuncturist is nationally certified. Well-trained acupuncturists usually check five pulses to determine weakened energy fields within the body while asking numerous questions. And generally, the use of fewer needles creates a more effective treatment, so ask if the acupuncturist uses numerous needles or few needles in their treatments.

Baths

Baths can be very effective in helping the body relax to induce sleep. Herbal baths are helpful in reducing pain and muscle tension, which ultimately results in a better night's sleep. Sage has been used for years as a remedy to relieve pain and to help induce restful sleep. Fresh sage leaves work best, so if you are inclined to grow your own, pick leaves before the plant begins to bloom. Place the leaves into a paper bag and store in a dark well-ventilated space until the leaves have dried. Once dried, store the dried leaves in a jar covered with paper. If you are not a gardener, sage found in bulk at a health food store or in the spice department of your favorite grocery store will do. Approximately five ounces of sage is needed for one bath. Heat a quart of water to boiling. Place the sage into a tea bag or coffee filter and put into the hot water. Let it steep for twenty-five minutes. Pour both the sage bag and the tea into the bath water as it is running, keeping the tea bag under the running water as best as possible. Periodically, squeeze the water out of the tea bag. Sage bath water should be as warm as possible, although, be sure it is not hot enough to scald or burn the body. Relax in the tea bath for twenty to twenty-five minutes. It may be necessary to have someone close by when stepping out of the bath, especially the first time or two that a sage bath is used. Many times pain is lessened and the body relaxed to the point of creating a feeling of weakness. After the bath, retire to bed and use the acupressure points for sleep.

Foods

Eating heavy or spicy foods before bed, or eating an excess of other foods and drinks during the day, may result in problems sleeping. Caffeine, tea, chocolate and soda are beverages that may tax the liver and gallbladder, waking the body between 11 PM and 3 AM. It is important to eat foods such as whole grains during the day as these foods promote the production of seratonin, a brain neurotransmitter that helps deepen sleep. The following are foods to eat and foods to avoid to promote deeper sleep.

Foods to Avoid

Coffee, tea, spicy foods, cola, chocolate, cigarettes, stimulant drugs, alcohol, refined carbohydrates, sugar, additives and preservatives.

Foods to Enjoy

Leafy, green vegetables, whole grains (other than wheat), fruit (mulberries and lemons calm the mind), cherries, tomato juice, brown rice, bananas and foods low in fat and cholesterol.

Herbal

Many herbs are helpful in relaxing the body in preparation for sleep. When accompanied with a sage bath and acupressure, herbs become even more effective in helping to bring about deep sleep. Drink herbal teas either during the sage bath or directly before a sage bath for best results.

Herbs Applied Topically

Nutmeg: Mix a fine paste of nutmeg and Ghee. Apply around the eyes and on your forehead for a beneficial treatment in helping you to fall asleep.

Herbs Taken As Teas

Teas made with the following herbs may be very helpful in promoting better sleep. Use one to two heaping teaspoons of dried herb per cup of hot water:

German Chamomile (Also helpful for congestion, eczema, colic, bites and stings, indigestion, mild asthma, morning sickness and sore nipples.)

Hops (Best for overactive minds, sedative, tension, aids in digestion, insomnia.) Can be mixed with chamomile in equal parts.

Lavender (Relieves muscle spasms, antidepressant, antiseptic, antibacterial and stimulates blood flow.) Sprinkling lavender oil on your pillow covering is also beneficial in promoting restful sleep.

Linden (Helpful for sinus headaches, calms the mind, reduces stress, calms feelings of panic, palpitations, nasal congestion, lowers high blood pressure and acts as a sedative.)

Licorice (Anti-inflammatory, expectorant, demulcent, adrenal agent, mild laxative, reduces stomach secretions while producing a protective mucous for the stomach, estrogenic, mild anti-arthritic, helpful for the liver and kidneys.)

Oats (Helpful in lowering cholesterol, improves stamina, nervous conditions, mild antidepressant, improves energy levels, relieves nervous exhaustion, reduces lethargy from multiple, chronic neurological pain, aids restful sleep.)

Passionflower (Helpful for lower backaches, mild sedative, insomnia, and pain relief.)

Siberian Ginseng (Insomnia)

Herbal Combinations

The following herbs can be mixed together in equal parts to help induce sleep:

Lady's Slipper Lady's Slipper is a rare herb, so may be very costly. (It is helpful as a sedative, and used in treating anxiety, stress-related disorders, palpitations, headaches, muscular tension, panic attacks, neurotic conditions, and calms the mind.)

Lemon Balm (Inhibits thyroid function, antiviral, calms the central nervous system, antispasmodic, relaxant and nervine.)

Skullcap (Also helpful to stimulate menstruation, mild nervine, relieve stress, anxiety attacks, sedative and relieves migraines.)

Valerian (Relaxant, mild sedative, encourages sleep, lower blood pressure, relieves anxiety, relieves muscle spasms.)

Nutritional Sleep Aids

Melatonin Is produced by the pineal gland when stimulated by sunlight. It is released at night to help regulate sleep. When taken supplemently, .3 mg to 1 mg per night is suggested.

Calcium Has a calming effect on the nervous system. It works together with magnesium in aiding in the contraction and relaxation of muscles including the heart. Take calcium, magnesium and zinc approximately 45 minutes before retiring to bed.

Magnesium Is a natural sedative aiding in the contraction and relaxation of muscles. Magnesium deficiency can cause insomnia.

Zinc Deficiency may be a factor in problematic sleep. When taken with calcium and magnesium, zinc enhances the effects of calcium and magnesium in helping with sleep problems.

Triptopan Is found in milk and poultry. Although, it is generally better to stay away from milk and milk products when suffering from fibromyalgia and chronic fatigue syndrome, poultry products may be consumed. The amino acid tryptopan converts to melatonin and can help induce sleep.

Apples or Apple Juice Contain malic acid which is believed to enhance the effects of magnesium. When taken before bedtime, apples also help stabilize the blood sugar through the night.

Massage

Massage may be very helpful in relaxing the body while releasing muscle tension and pain. It is important to drink plenty of water before and after a massage to help move toxins released by the massage out of the body. A warm bath that induces sweating is also helpful for releasing toxins.

Shiatsu treatments used during massage are very effective in deeply relaxing the body, thereby promoting deep sleep. Many well-trained massage therapists practice shiatsu, a form of Japanese acupressure.

Warm oil massage using warm sesame rubbed on the scalp and soles of the feet is an effective way to induce sleep.

Mind/Body

Listening to soft or meditative music thirty minutes before retiring to bed each night can serve as a signal to the mind and body to begin relaxing. There are also numerous yoga exercises designed to help relax the mind and body in preparation for sleep.

Other

Allowing natural sunlight into the eyes without the use of sunglasses or colored contact lenses may help deepen sleep. According to Dr. William Kellas, in his book Thriving in a Toxic World, colored contact lenses and sunglasses interfere with melatonin syntheses, decreasing the amount of melatonin produced by the body. This problem may be exacerbated when working night shifts. If sleep time is during the day rather than at night, a daytime sleep schedule does not allow enough time for sunlight to enter the eyes, once again interfering with the melatonin syntheses.

Natural Pain Aids

The agonizing effect that pain from FMS and CFS has on the body can be debilitating. The following information may help you alleviate some, if not all, of it.

Stretching exercises loosen muscles, helping to diminish pain. There may be a number of exercise programs available in your area. I would caution against using any aerobic exercises as even low impact and mild aerobics can be hard on the body until it is strong and nutritionally sound. Water aerobics may be helpful, although, if chlorine is used for cleansing the water, the affects of chlorine on the body may cause more harm than good. If your pool is treated with chlorine, ask the manager to switch to a non-toxic treatment. This not only benefits those with arthritis and fibromyalgia, but everyone else who comes in contact with the water.

Walking is another exercise which is very helpful in treating pain and fatigue. Although, according to Dr. Joe Elrod if you feel worse after exercising that may be an indication that you suffer from nutritional deficiencies. It is important to use a pure nutritional product for at least two weeks before beginning large muscle exercises, such as walking; thus allowing nutrients to build up in the muscle which supports their activity.

Herbs may also be beneficial in alleviating or diminishing painful symptoms. Many of them can be grown in your garden or sourced through your local health food store or grocery store. Herbs are most generally more effective when used in a more natural form such as in teas or salads, as processing many times will lessen their potency. Following are some herbs that worth a try:

Lavender - Can be effective in relieving muscle spasms.

Linden - Is helpful for sinus headaches.

Licorice - Is an anti-inflammatory, so it can be effective in helping with mild arthritic pain.

Oats – Have been found to be effective in controlling chronic neurological pain.

Passionflower - Has been found to be useful for lower backaches and general pain relief.

Lemon Balm - Is useful in that it inhibits thyroid function, is an antispasmodic, relaxant and nervine.

Skullcap - Is helpful to relieve stress, anxiety attacks, and migraines.

Valerian - Can help with muscle spasms, as it is a relaxant and mild sedative.

Sugar, processed foods and caffeine may promote muscle and joint pain. Many times eliminating these foods from the diet will help diminish pain within a matter of a few days. Preservatives may also contribute to pain.

Another suggestion, although you will have to pay for their services, is that it is quite effective to receive a massage or chiropractic treatments. Then follow up with a sage (see section on "Sleep Aids") or Epsom salts bath.

Finally, two effective treatments for pain, when used on a regular basis, are acupuncture and acupressure. Acupressure, since it can be self-administered, is quite cost effective. And the more it is used, the quicker its effects for pain are noticed. When I first began using acupressure, it may have taken from ten to fifteen minutes to feel the effects, although, as I used it more regularly, the less time its effects took. Today, a short thirty seconds to two minutes of acupressure eliminates most pain symptoms.

The following pages contain numerous acupressure treatments which are helpful for specific symptoms related to fibromyalgia and chronic fatigue syndrome. Use them as often as necessary.

Acupressure Points

1. Deep Breathing is very important to do to revitalize and purify the body. It is also important to breath deeply before beginning the acupressure treatments to achieve optimum results.

2. As I have mentioned in other areas of this book, all treatments in this book are treatments I've used on myself and my daughter for relief from the symptoms of FMS. This book is not intended as a substitute for medical advice from your physician. The reader should consult with his or her physician with any questions of health and/or symptoms that may require medical attention or diagnosis.

3. In doing acupressure on specific points, place a finger on the point and, without removing the finger, move it in three circular motions. Then gently press the area for one to three minutes.

4. The amount of pressure depends on the individual. If you experience pain, gently reduce pressure until you find a balance between pain and pleasure.

5. Acupressure is not intended to increase your tolerance for pain, discontinue pressing an area that is extremely painful.

6. Many times when you press on one point, you may feel pain in another part of the body. That pain indicates that those areas are related.

7. If your hands are in pain or too weak to use, knuckles, avocado pits, a golf ball or pencil eraser may be used to press on the points.

8. Shoulders and upper back will need more pressure than other parts of the body.

9. A good massage therapist can stimulate areas you are not able to reach. My husband also tries to give me a firm back or foot massage two to four times per week, especially when I have tension and know my sleep will be affected by that tension.

10. Learn the points and their corresponding symptoms. You will then have a useful technique that will help control symptoms anytime they arise.

Headache or Neck-Head Pain Acupressure Points

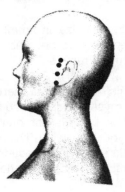 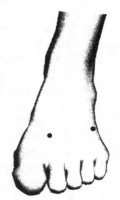

A. Location is one-half inch above the front of the depression in front of the ear which deepens when mouth is open.

B. Location is directly in front of the ear opening in a depression which deepens when mouth is open.

C. Location is one-half inch below depression in B.

D. Location is the indention behind the earlobe.

E. Location at the top of the foot in the valley between the big toe and the second toe.

F. Located on top of the foot, one inch above the webbing of the fourth and fifth toes in the groove between the bones.

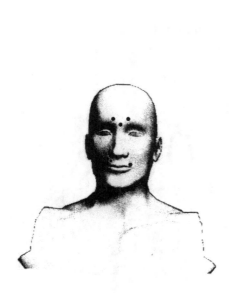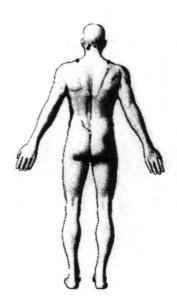

A. Location is in the indentations on either side of the bridge of the nose where the eyebrows meet the bridge of the nose.
B. Location is right in the middle where the bridge meets the fore-head.
C. Location is at the bottom of the cheekbone, below the pupil of the eye.
D. Location in the center of the back of the head in a hollow under the base of the skull.
E. Location is below the base of the skull between the two vertical neck muscles.
F. Located about one and one-half inches below the base of the skull, on the vertical muscles.
G. Located on the highest point of the shoulder muscle, one to two inches from the side of the lower neck. (Pregnant women should press this point lightly.)

Acupressure Points For Hip, Leg And Foot Pain

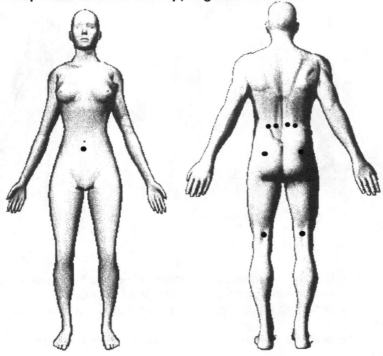

A. Location is two finger widths directly below the belly button.
B. (Be sure not to press on any disintegrating disks or fractures or broken bones.) Located in the lower back, two finger widths away from the spine at the waist level.
C. Located in the lower back, four finger widths away from the spine at the waist level.
D. Located one to two finger widths out side the large bone in the base of the spine.
E. Located in the center of the back of the knee.

Acupressure Points For Shoulder, Arm, Hand, Middle and Upper Back Pain

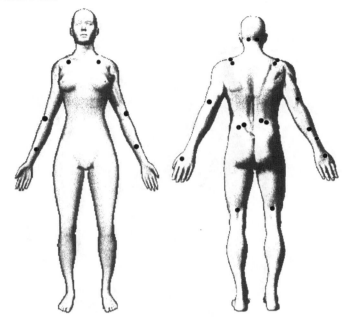

A. Located four finger widths up from the armpit crease in the outer part of the chest, and one finger width inward.

B. Located on the inner wrist two and one-half finger widths up the arm from the center of the inner wrist.

C. Location is below the base of the skull between the two vertical neck muscle.

D. Located on the highest point of the shoulder muscle, one to two inches from the side of the lower neck. (pregnant women should press lightly on this point.).

E. Located one inch below and one-half inch to the center of D.

F. Located in the center of the outer arm approximately one-third of the way down between the shoulder and the elbow where the upper arm muscle ends.

G. Located on the upper edge of the elbow crease.

H. Located two and one-half finger widths above the wrist crease on the outer forearm midway between the two bones of the arm.

I. Located in the webbing between the thumb and the index finger. (Pregnant women should not use this point.)

J. The waist points are located in the lower back two and four widths away from the spine at the waist level.

K. Located in the center of the back of the knee in the crease.

Acupressure Points To Boost the Immune System

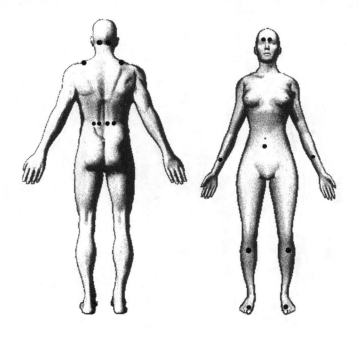

A. Location is below the base of the skull between the two vertical neck muscles.

B. Location is on the highest point on the shoulder muscle, one to two inches from the side of the lower neck.

C. Location in the lower back, two and four finger widths away from the spine at the waist level.

D. Location in the indentations on either side of the bridge of the nose where the eyebrows meet the bridge of the nose.

E. Two and one-half finger widths up the arm from the center of the inner wrist crease, midway between the two forearm bones.

F. Three fingers widths below the belly button.

G. Four fingers widths below the kneecap, and one finger width on the outside of the shinbone. A muscle should flex as you move your feet up and down if you are on the right spot.

H. In the valley between the big toe and the second toe on the top of the feet.

Acupressure Points for Sleep

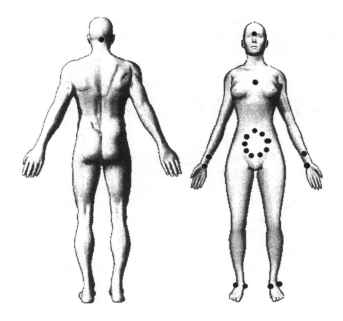

A. Location is in the center of the back of the head in a hollow under the base of the skull.

B. Located on the inner wrist two and one-half finger widths up the arm from the center of the inner wrist.

C. Located on the crease of the wrist toward the palm area of the hand.

D. Location begins four finger widths below the belly button. Continue at one o'clock, two o'clock, etc. around in a circle on the abdomen, pressing one inch inside of the hip bone structure and one inch above the pelvic bone.

E. The point on the inside of the heel located below the inside of the anklebone in a slight indentation.

F. The point located on the outside of the heel located in the indentation directly below the anklebone.

G. Located directly below the eyebrows at the bridge of the nose.

Shopping For Foods

Perhaps one of the most commonly asked asked questions at my seminars is; "How do you shop?" What they are really asking is; "When I start to purchase products for myself, what is considered to be 'good,' and what isn't?" This chapter will deal with that question in a straight forward, practical way. Obviously, all foods can not be reviewed, but enough of them can be addressed to give you a flying start. So here are some tips, and a list featuring my own rating system, (Best, Not Good, etc.):

1. Organic foods would be my choice as the best source of foods, but they are not absolutely necessary.
2. Always clean or soak fruits and vegetables in a solution to take preservative chemicals off of the outside of the food.
3. Always choose "fresh" or "closest to nature", when purchasing foods. A general rule of thumb would be this: If the food looks close to its natural state, it should be more nutritional. If the food doesn't resemble the grain or food it originated from, it may be too processed and would have less nutritional value. Foods closest to nature are generally found in the outer perimeters of the store, so this is where I do the majority of my grocery shopping. Exceptions to this would be cereals and in some stores, frozen foods.
4. If your local food store does not carry some of the foods rated as "Best," check into a local health food co-op as they may have them available. If there are no co-ops in your area, try one of the mail order suppliers found in the back of this book.

The following is a partial list of common foods:

A. CEREALS — Choose cereals that are non-wheat based, processed very little and have 5 or less gm. of sugars per serving. Check the ingredients on the side of the package. If the first few ingredients are wheat, corn syrup, fructose, etc., these would not be good choices. Always choose cereals that are high in fiber (2 or more gm. per serving).

Choices:
Boxed Cereals — **Not Acceptable.** (Check side panel for nutritional information listed above, you may find a few that would meet the criteria listed above.)
Rolled Oats — (Old Fashioned or Steel Cut) **Best**
9 - 12 - or 15 Grain Cereals (Cooked) — **Best**

Gluten Free Cereals— **Best**
Other "Wheat Free", less processed cereals may be okay. Check the sides of the box for the amount of sugar and to make sure the cereal is not made from wheat.
Rice — **Best**

B. BREADS & PASTAS
Try to find breads that are made from grains other than wheat. Enriched processed wheat flour is the same as wheat flour. For more information on common grains used in breads see in the flour section of this book.

Choices:
White or Wheat breads — **Not Good**
9+ Grain Breads — **Not Good** (Although, this bread would be better than breads that are entirely wheat based as it has less wheat, it is still better to stay away from wheat until the body is completely healthy.)
Bagels — **Not Good.**
English Muffins — **Not Good.**
Soft Shell Tacos — **Generally OK**
Rice Breads — **Best**
Semolina or Other Grain Breads — **Best**

PASTAS - Stay away from most wheat pastas. Health food stores have pastas made from grains other than wheat, as well as pastas made from semolina flour. Generally, pastas made from semolina flour, have a consistency and flavor very similar to pastas made from wheat. (Semolina is a meal made from the hard kearnels of wheat.)
Note: When baking and cooking pastas and breads, I make twice as much as needed and freeze half for later use. This makes future meals much quicker and less messy. To heat pastas, I let them set on the counter until they are thawed, then heat them by adding them to a casserole dish.

C. VEGETABLES and FRUITS—When purchasing fruits and   vegetables, purchase fresh first. If fresh is not available, choose frozen (without sugars or sweeteners or preservatives added). The last choice of vegetables and fruits would be canned. The only exception to that rule would be in the case of dried beans and potatoes as they release more vitamins and minerals after they are cooked.

D. MEATS — Organic is always best, although if buying organic is too expensive for you, other meats may be used. Antibiotics, steroids and other chemicals in the feed which is fed to livestock may create digestive problems for you when ingesting meat. To determine if the meat you eat is causing stress on your body, do a simple pulse test. To pulse test, take your pulse one minute before eating meat, 20 minutes after eating the meat and then one hour later. If the pulse rises on the second check, your body may be indicating a sensitivity to that food. The higher the rise in pulse, the greater the sensitivity. (Obviously, this test can be used to check for sensitivity to any food.)

Fresh Meats — **Best**
Pre-Cooked — **Not Good** (May contain preservatives, read ingredient labels to be sure there are no preservatives.)
Fish — Fresh or Frozen **Best**
      Canned **Generally OK**
Luncheon Meats, Hot Dogs, Sausages, Bacon — **Not Good**
Sliced Meats From a Deli — Check for preservatives:
      Without Preservatives — **Best**
      With Preservatives – **Not Good**

TVP (Texturized Vegetable Protein) This product, made from soybeans, and can be blended with ground beef, chicken, or fish, or used as a substitute for ground beef, chicken or fish. It comes in chunks (chicken or fish), or in a ground consistency, (ground beef). When using with ground beef, use half TVP and half ground beef. Reconstitute TVP using equal amounts of hot water. Let set to reconstitute for approximately 10 minutes before adding to beef.

E. BEANS & LENTILS — These foods, containing numerous vitamins and minerals, are high in protein and are an excellent source of fiber.

Dried — **Best**
Canned — **Best**

F. CANNED SOUPS — Check for preservatives, and choose those that have little or no preservatives in them. This source of food, when purchased in cans in the grocery store would be a **Poor** choice of food.

Home-Made Soups — **Best**
Soups Canned In Jars – **Generally OK**

G. PACKAGED MEALS

Boxed, Packaged Foods/Meals — **Not Good**
Frozen, Packaged Foods/Meals — **Generally OK** to **Not Good**
(Look for preservatives, check ingredients and nutritional content of frozen dinners.)

H. MILK

Whole, Skim or Part Skim From Cows — **Generally Not Good**
(Many people with FMS/CFS are sensitive to, or allergic to cows milk.)
Goat Milk – **Best**
Soy (Plain), Rice (Plain), Oat (Plain) — **Best**
Soy (Vanilla or Chocolate), Rice (Vanilla or Chocolate),
Oat (Vanilla or Chocolate) — **Not Good**

I. BUTTERS

Real Butter — **Generally Ok** (Use sparingly in case there are sensitivities to milk products.)
Rice Butter — **Best**
Other Artificial Margarines or Spreads — **Not Good**

J. CHEESE AND SOUR CREAMS — It is best to stay away from traditional cheeses and sour creams made out of cows milk due to allergies or sensitivities to milk products. If you do choose to use regular cheese, it is best to choose white rather than yellow or cheese. (Colored cheeses many times have artificial colorings in them.)

Yellow or Colored Cheese — **Not Good**
Soy or Rice Cheeses — **Best**
Soy or Rice Sour Creams — **Best**

K. CONDIMENTS —When used sparingly, condiments are okay. It is best to buy soy or rice based mayonnaise and dressings whenever possible. Regular ketchup and barbecue sauce in small amounts would be acceptable.

L. SUGARS — The goal is to work refined sugars out of the diet. For more information refer to the section on sweeteners.

Stevia — **Best**
Fructose — Use only at the beginning to help in cutting refined sugars out of the diet. (See section on "Sweeteners".)
Maple Syrup & Honey — **Not Good**

Corn Syrups — **Not Good**

Jams & Jellies — Purchase only "all fruit" types. Check for added sugars.

White or Brown Sugars — **Not Good**

M. CHOCOLATE — Substitute *unsweetened* carob for chocolate. Substitute *unsweetened* carob chips for chocolate chips. Use stevia to sweeten carob.

N. ICE CREAM — Due to the fact most sufferers of FMS/CFS are sensitive to milk, milk products and sugar, ice cream is not a good source of food for them as they may cause adverse symptoms. Rather than purchasing ice cream, purchase frozen, unsweetened fruit, tofu, and a choice of milk listed earlier in this section. Blend milk, tofu, frozen fruit, vanilla and stevia together in a blender and use in place of ice cream.

O. CHIPS — Chips are a poor source of nutrition. When purchasing chips for a special occasion, buy only "baked" chips, as they have a much lower content of fats. Use plicate sauce for dip, or create your own dip using spices in tofu, or non-cow milk sour cream.

P. MEXICAN, ITALIAN, OR CHINESE FOODS — **Avoid Boxed Mixes.**

Mexican — Create your own meals rather than using box or package mixes. Purchase refried beans, soft tortilla shells and add fresh vegetables in burritos and tacos. Use salsa, picante sauce, etc. for condiments.

Italian — Source pastas other than wheat pastas. Use vegetables sautéed in olive oil and add spices for toppings.

Chinese —Stir fry your own vegetables and add your own sauces. Whole and long grain rice is always wonderful, nutritious, and is a great source of carbohydrates.

Q. POTATOES

Fresh — **Best**

Instant — **Not Good**

Frozen — **Generally OK** (If there are no preservatives in them.)

Bagged, Ready to Heat Up — **Generally OK**

R. OILS — Use olive oil or real butter for cooking. Use vegetable oils only in foods where the oils are not being heated.

GENERAL INFORMATION:

> Try to keep sugar to 5 gm./serving or less when purchasing foods.

> When baking with flours other than traditional processed, enriched wheat flour, use equal amounts of soda as baking powder.

> LAUNDRY PRODUCTS — Use only environmentally safe laundry and cleaning products.
Whitening, Bleaching & Disinfecting Products – Use only environmentally safe products.

Flours and Grains

Grains have been around almost since the beginning of time. Many of our grains are some of the same grains used by the original colonists of the United States, although the processing of these grains have made baking and cooking with them quite different from the times of early settlers. As one becomes more knowledgeable about the different grains, it becomes obvious why grains were and continue to be such an important part of daily diets. In getting well and maintaining a healthy body it has been very important for me to omit processed white flours from my diet. The next few pages will tell about many of the grains that have replaced white processed flour in our cupboards. Most of these grains can be found in local health food stores, and if they are not available, the stores will know how and where to source them.

Knowing and understanding the different forms of flours and how they work has been helpful in baking with them since baking with flours other than processed white flours can change the size and texture of baked goods. To begin, let's take a look at refined white flour. During the process of refining the wheat to create the white flour we know so well and use in the majority of our baking, wheat loses up to 80% of its nutrients. Enriched white flour has only four of the sixteen nutrients of what nature intended. And during the process of bleaching the flour, essential amino acids or the protein part of the flour is also destroyed.

Some flours also contain gluten or protein that controls the bread's ability to raise. Gluten-containing grains in descending order are wheat, spelt, kamut, rye, oats and barley. According to the Rodale Research Center in eastern Pennsylvania, all grains contain some gluten, although those with a very low amount of gluten are considered gluten free. Gluten free grains are corn, millet, buckwheat, amaranth, quinoa, rice, sorghum and teff.

Grains and flours can become rancid if kept at improper temperatures. To avoid this from happening, it is helpful when buying flours in bulk to store them in the freezer in glass jars. Be sure to allow the flour to come to room temperature for best results in baking.

Types of Grains and Flours
Kamut

Kamut, which originated in the Nile region of Egypt, has never been crossbred. The kamut grain contains more proteins, lipids and measures 88 percent higher in minerals than common wheat. Kamut wheat contains more gluten so if a person is sensitive to gluten, this would be a grain/flour to avoid. Many times those who are sensitive to wheat find kamut flour to be a good substitute. Kamut has a buttery taste and is much higher in nutritional value than most other grains, containing approximately 30 percent more protein than other wheats. It is also much higher in amino acids and fatty acids. Kamut flour can be used for almost any baking needs you would use wheat flour in, although, due to its color, baked goods generally come out browner. For measurements to substitute kamut wheat for whole-wheat flour see the "Substitutions" section in this chapter.

Spelt

Spelt grain is easily digested, therefore it may be a good grain for those of us who suffer with digestive disturbances. Originating in Asia, spelt contains many of the nutrients and amino acids necessary for a healthy body, therefore it is a grain that is good to keep around for baking needs. This grain, which is very disease resistant, has its own protective covering called a husk or hull, which guards the spelt grain against outside pollutants. This protective husk, which must be removed before the grain is used, protects the spelt grain during the growing process and in storage. Although the spelt grain has more of a buttery flavor than wheat grain, it can be used in place of wheat flour in cooking and baking. I have found spelt to be a great flour substitute for white processed flour. The baked goods come out with similar consistency as they would with processed flour, and many times the buttery flavor can be noticed, adding a wonderful addition to baked goods.

Oat

For those who have high cholesterol or high blood sugar, oat flour can be a very healthy substitute for wheat flour. It has been found that oats help to lower cholesterol, regulate blood sugar, reduce chances of getting certain cancers and push poisonous wastes through your system fast. Oats are a highly nutritious grain that is low in saturated fat, low in cholesterol and has been found to help reduce the risk of heart disease. It is a grain that grows on a stalk similar to the wheat grain. Oat flour seems to add more moisture to cakes and breads, making it "heavier," than wheat. If this flour is difficult to find in your area, it can be made by putting "rolled oats" into a blender and blending until it is of flour consistency.

Amaranth

Amaranth originated with the Aztecs in Mexico and South America as well as in China and was once considered to be a very important grain and daily staple for health. Today it can be found in Midwestern states such as Kansas and Nebraska. The seeds of the amaranth plant can be eaten, cooked, or ground into flour for baking uses. This source of flour is very nutritious, as it is a good source of vegetable protein, amino acids, lysine, vitamins and minerals. Due to the lack of gluten in amaranth flour, a gluten product such as potato starch, cornstarch, tapioca starch or soy flour needs to be added in many recipes. This gluten-free plant is related to the pigweed family so in many cases can be used as a substitute by those who are allergic to grains. Once purchased, this grain is best stored in the freezer. If not stored properly this flour can develop a strong odor, becoming rancid or bitter.

Barley

Barley is a cereal grass native to Asia and Ethiopia. Its leaves have become a popular source of antioxidants and its phytochemical properties are recommended by natural healers. Barley contains a large proportion of carbohydrates and protein and was used in years past to help conserve wheat by replacing part of the wheat flour in recipes with barley flour. Barley flour has a strong flavor so generally would be used with another grain in baking.

Buckwheat

Buckwheat is a grain that provides the highest source of protein in the plant kingdom, higher than that of soybeans. In comparing the protein content in buckwheat to that of beef, there is as much protein in two pounds of buckwheat as is in one pound of beef. The amino acids found in buckwheat allow the protein in it to be used by our bodies in the most efficient way possible. It is native to the shores of the Caspian Sea and was introduced into Western Europe during the 16th century. The seeds, which are ground into flour are tiny, black and have three-corners. The buckwheat plant is actually a fruit since it has seeds and is closely related to the rhubarb plant. It is usually grown organically and is a great source of vitamins, minerals and dietary fiber. It has also been found to be helpful in preventing atherosclerosis. It is a fat and cholesterol free food. Twenty percent of our suggested daily fiber intake can be found in one cup of ground buckwheat. Buckwheat can be used as a flour in griddlecakes and some breads or it can be eaten as a cooked cereal.

Corn

Corn flour is made from whole kernels of corn that are finely ground. This flour comes in white or yellow depending on the color of the corn used to make the flour. It is used in combination with other flours in baked goods or is used for breading for meats or in vegetables. Corn contains gluten, so should be avoided when a person is gluten intolerant.

Quinoa

Quinoa has been grown in the South American Andes since at least 3,000 BC. Ancient Inca Indians revered it as a "sacred" grain, and today's research has suggested this grain comes as close to having all of the essential life sustaining nutrients as any other food source in the vegetable or animal kingdoms. There are about 2,000 varieties of Quinoa with colors ranging from off-white to black. It is high in protein, vitamins E and B, and is high in calcium, phosphorous, and iron. The bitter coating on the seeds called saponin, acts as a natural insect and bird repellent. This coating forms a soapy solution in water and seeds must be washed two or three times before eating the seed to remove the bitter taste it produces. This seed, which is high in oil and fat, can be cooked very quickly for a fast, hot cereal or the flour can be made into muffins or pancakes.

Rice

Rice is a grain found in the grass family and is gluten free. Due to its popularity, it is the second most produced food in the world and comes in many varieties. It is a natural source of vitamin B and although it originated in Southeast Asia, China and India it can be found growing around the world. Rice flour has a drier consistency and leaves a "grainier" taste when used in cooking. It is a very good alternative flour to be used in place of other white flours. Varieties include; Brown rice, sweet brown rice, basmati, texmati, calmatil and other "specialty" forms.

Soy

Soy flour is made from soybeans that have been roasted and ground into a powder. Soy flour has a long shelf life, up to twelve months. It can be found in either a full-fat form, which contains the natural oils found in the soybean or in a low-fat form, which has the oils removed. It is an excellent source of protein, iron, vitamin B and calcium and isoflavones, which can help prevent certain chronic diseases such as cancer, heart disease and osteoporosis. Low-fat soy flour is also a good source of fiber. Eggs can be substituted for in a recipe by replacing one egg with one-tablespoon soy flour and one tablespoon water. Products baked with soy flour may brown sooner, so the oven temperature should be lowered slightly during baking. It should be stirred before measuring it since it tends to pack down in the container.

Refined Flours

Refined flours made from wheat

Refined flours may carry a number of different names including all-purpose flour, bread flour, self-rising flour, cake flour and pastry flour. To better understand these flours and the differences that occur during processing let's take a look at the nutritional content of whole grains versus their refined flours.

Calorie content of refined flour made from wheat actually increases about ten percent because everything else has been taken out. Approximately 66% of the B vitamins, 70% of all minerals and an average of 19% of protein have been removed. Fiber content has decreased about 79%. Except for the carbohydrates, most nutritional value has been removed from refined flours. Buckwheat flour does not seem to be significantly harmed by the refinement, retaining approximately 85 to 100% of its nutrients.

Let's take a look at those flours that have been fortified with vitamins and their nutritional content. Two nutrients that have been removed during processing, vitamins B6 and folic acid, are not replaced. Of the nine minerals removed from processed flours, only three (calcium, phosphorus and iron) are sometimes replaced in fortified flours. Be sure to check the label to be sure these three have been fortified in the flour. Many of the vitamins and minerals that are replaced in processed, fortified flours, have undergone a processing that leaves them in a state in which our digestive systems will have a very low absorption rate. When we eat refined flours we are eating a very nutrient poor food, far from the wheat and its nutrients intended by nature.

Refined meals made from corn

During the refinement process cornmeal loses much less of its nutritional content than wheat flours since it goes through much less. The refinement process doesn't harm it significantly, although the biggest drawback is the oils becoming rancid if the meal isn't freshly ground making them less nutritious. Grinding fresh corn for corn meal is delicious compared to cornmeal found on grocery shelves.

Substitutions

To have a smoother texture when baking with rice flour, the Rice Council of America suggests mixing the rice flour with the liquid called for in a recipe. Bring to a boil, then cool before adding other ingredients.

Also, according to the Rice Council of America, coarse flours do not need to be sifted before measuring; however, they need more leavening than wheat flour. For each cup of coarse flour, use 2 1/2 tsp. of baking powder.

These are the substitutions recommended by the Rice Council of America.

For 1 cup of wheat flour substitute:
    3/4 c. sweet rice flour
    1 scant c. corn meal (fine)
    1 c. corn flour
    5/8 c. potato starch flour
    3/4 c. corn meal

These are other wheat flour substitutions. For 1 cup of wheat flour, substitute the following:
    1 c. amaranth flour
    1 c. millet flour
    1 1/3 c. oat flour
    1 1/4 c. rye flour
    7/8 c. kamut flour
    1 c. spelt flour
    7/8 c. buckwheat flour
    1 1/3 c. barely flour
    3/4 c. garbanzo bean (chickpea) or other bean flours
    1 c. quinoa
    1/2 c. so + 1/2 c. potato starch

Substitutes for 1 cup whole-wheat flour include:
    1 c. kamut flour
    1 c. spelt flour (reduce amount of liquid by 25%)

To replace 1 Tbsp. of wheat flour as a thickener use:
    1 1/2 tsp. arrowroot
    1 Tbsp. oat flour
    1 Tbsp. brown or white rice flour
    1 1/2 tsp. cornstarch
    2 tsp. tapioca
    1 Tbsp. brown or white rice flour

Sweeteners

Since eliminating sugars played such a vital role in regaining in my health it was important to learn more about the sweeteners available in our markets. Studies have shown each person eats between 35 and 150 teaspoons of sugar per day, which adds up to 65 to 100 pounds (cane or beet) sugar and 79 pounds of other (like honey) sweeteners per year. Since sugar provides "empty" calories, it is not surprising that many Americans have problems with obesity. Another surprising statistic is the 16 pounds of artificial or chemical sweeteners consumed by Americans each year. Sweeteners may be the cause of health problems ranging from kidney damage to allergies to cancer. Sugars have no natural fiber or nutrition!

The more "natural" sweeteners may seem to contain more vitamins and minerals, although, through commercial processing these sweeteners can lose much of their vitamin content. For instance, commercially processed honeys may lose between 33%-50% of their original vitamin content.

Sweeteners, What are they?

Glucose is sometimes called dextrose or blood sugar. Fructose is found naturally in fruits and honey and is a simple sugar. Lactose comes from milk, better know as "milk" sugar. Sucrose is a mixture of fructose and glucose. Maltose occurs naturally in sprouted grain. Let's take a look at number of sugars and sweetners:

Brown Rice Syrup: Brown rice syrup is made from slow cooking brown rice until it develops into a thick, sweet syrup. It has been a traditional Asian sweetener for many years and is considered to be a complex sugar. It is interchangeable with honey in cooking and baking.

Barley Malt: Barley Malt syrup is milder than blackstrap molasses and not as sweet as honey. This syrup enters the bloodstream slowly and offers trace amounts of B vitamins and several minerals. This sweetener is made from sprouted, roasted barley grain and has a sweet nutty flavor. It comes in granular form or syrup.

Fructose: Fructose is the sugar derived from fruit and closely resembles white sugar. It is twice as sweet as white sugar, so 1/2 as much can be used as white sugar. It breaks down more slowly in the body than sugar and does not provide any nutritional benefits.

150

Date Sugar: Date sugar is made from ground dehydrated dates; therefore, it is actually not a sugar. It is high in vitamins and minerals and has a high concentration of naturally occurring sugars. This "sugar" doesn't dissolve well but is good for cooking and baking.

Fruit Juice Sweetener: This sweetener goes through very little processing and is generally made from juices of pineapple, pear, peach or clarified grape juice.

Honey: Honey is primarily glucose, a simple sugar. Commercially processed, clarified honey looses from 33% to 50% of its original vitamin content. Raw honey contains one of the highest enzyme contents of all foods and in its raw state has many minerals. The flavor of honey varies with the flower used to make it. Some of the types of honey one might find on the store shelves would be buckwheat, clover, orange blossom, wildflower and sage. Each has a flavor all its own and is delicious to use in many ways.

Maple Syrup: This syrup is made from boiling down the sap from the maple tree and is mainly sucrose, a simple sugar. Maple syrup is classified in grade by its color, the lighter the color, the lighter the flavor. Maple syrup adds a wonderful flavor to baked goods.

Molasses: Molasses is formed from the liquid spun out of cane sugar during processing. It is graded by color and consists of 20-25% water, 50% sucrose, 10% ash, and includes some protein and organic acids. It is rich in iron and vitamin B6, calcium and potassium. Organic unsulphured molasses is best for optimal quality.

Sorghum: Sorghum, a grain related to millet, is processed into a sweetener by crushing the stocks and boiling the extracted juice into syrup. It is lighter and milder than molasses.

Sucanat: Sucanat contains more vitamins, minerals and other trace nutrients than sugar cane. It is made from the dehydrated juice of the organic sugar cane and is about 88% sucrose or simple sugar, as compared to table sugar which is 99% sucrose. It has a flavor that is similar to a very mild molasses flavor and can be used in most cooking and baking.

Stevia: Stevia comes from an herb and is about 10-15 times sweeter than regular sugar. This wonderful sweetener contains nearly 100 identified phytonutrients and volatile oils. Since stevia is much sweeter than sugar, the amounts consumed to sweeten food make the nutritive benefits very little. Research has shown stevia may actually lower blood sugar levels, making it a natural substitute that can be used by diabetics. For many years, stevia has been grown overseas and in the past few years it has been grown in gardens in the United States, making it a very accessible and inexpensive sweetener to have in one's cupboards.

Turbinado: Turbinado comes from molasses during the first separation in processing. It is identical to white sugar in the way it is absorbed.

In working toward eliminating sugars from the diet, the following chart may be helpful in making substitutions. These measurements are equal to 1 cup of sugar:

Sweetener	Source	To Replace 1c. Sugar	Liquid Reduction
Brown rice syrup	Brown rice	1 cup	1/4 cup
Fructose	Corn or beet	1/2 cup	3/4 cup
Date sugar	Dates	2/3 cup	—-
Barley malt	Barley	1 cup	1/4 cup
Fruit juice	Fruit	1 cup	1/8 cup
Honey	Bees	1/2 cup	1/4 cup
Maple syrup	Maple tree	1/2-1/3 cup	—-
Molasses	Sugar cane	1/2 cup	1/4 cup
Sorghum	Sorghum	1/2 cup	1/4 cup
Sucanat	Organic cane	1 cup	—-
Stevia (powder)	Herb	1 tsp.	—-
Stevia (liquid)	Herb	10 drops	—-
Turbinado	Sugar cane	1 cup	—-

RECIPES

Breads and Desserts

Almond Cluster
1 pkg. unsweetened carob chips
Olive oil to make carob creamy
Melt in double broiler.
1 1/2 c. slivered almonds
1/2 tsp. powdered stevia
Mix stevia with almonds. Pour into carob. Drop onto wax paper.

Blueberry Muffins
1 c. oat flour
3/4 c. rice flour
1/2 c. Soy Protein (vanilla)
1 1/2 c. Fiber Plan Daily Crunch
¼ tsp. xantham gum
1/2 tsp. salt
1 1/4 tsp. baking soda
1 1/4 tsp. baking powder
2 c. frozen blueberries
1/2 c. chopped nuts
3/4 tsp. stevia
2 c. soy or rice milk
1 egg (lightly beaten)
2 Tbsp. oil
Preheat oven to 350 degrees. In a large bowl, mix all the dry ingredients first before adding the nuts and fruits. In a separate bowl, mix together all the liquid ingredients. Then slowly add the liquid mixture to the dry ingredients until all blended together. Pour the batter into greased muffin pans (2/3 of the way up) and bake them for 25 minutes. A great snack to pack for the road or even to have on hand for unexpected company.

Bread Machine White Bread (Rose Moyers)
¾ cup water (90 ° to 100 °)
3 ¼ cups spelt flour
1 ½ tsp. salt
1 packet active dry yeast
¼ cup rice milk (90° to 100°)
1 tsp. sugar (needed for yeast)
2 tbsp. butter

Add liquid ingredients to pan. Add dry ingredients, except yeast to pan. Level ingredients, push some into corners of pan. Cut butter in 4 pieces and place in corners of pan. Make a well in center of dry ingredients: add yeast. Lock pan into bread maker. Program for Basic/Specialty and desired bread color. Start bread maker. When done, remove bread from pan and cool on rack.

Carob Almond Cookies
1/3 c. almond butter
1 1/2 large apples
1/4 tsp. baking powder
1 1/4 c. brown rice flour
3/4 carob powder
1/4 tsp. salt
2 Tbsp. oil
2 eggs
30 almonds
Puree all liquids in blender until smooth. Add all powder and mix. Add nuts. Drop spoonful on baking sheet. Bake 10-12 minutes.

Vanilla Tofu Ice Cream
2 lbs. Tofu
2 c. soy milk
1 c. oil
1 tsp. stevia
6 Tbsp. vanilla protein
2 Tbsp. vanilla
1/4 tsp. salt
Blend all the ingredients until smooth in a blender or food processor. Freeze the mixture in a hand-operated or electric ice cream maker and serve.

Coconut Mud BonBons
1/4 c. figs (chopped)
3/4 c. dates (chopped)
1/2 c. unsweetened coconut
3/4 c. shredded english walnuts
1/4 c. Shaklee Soy Protein
1/4 tsp. powdered stevia
 Mix together in a bowl and add:
1/2 c. soy nut butter
1/2 c. peanut butter (without sugar)
Mix butter into above mixture with hands. Roll into small balls. Coat with shredded coconut. Chill before serving.

Cool Lime Cheesecake
Crust:
2 1/4 c. cracker crumb
1/3 c. sugar
1/2 c. butter melted
Filling:
20 g. fat free cream cheese (15 oz.)
1 tsp. stevia
5 oz. tofu
1 c. sour cream
3 Tbsp. oat flour
3 eggs
2/3 c. lime juice
1 tsp. vanilla
Bake at 325 degrees for 50-55 minutes. Cool 1 hour. Refrigerate over night.

EZ Carob Fudge
1 1/2 c. peanut butter (no sugar added)
6 s. unsweetened carob
1/2 c. dates (diced)
1/2 silvered almonds
1 tsp. vanilla
1/2 c. soy milk
1/2 c., rice sweetener
1 tsp. stevia
Combine carob chips and peanut butter. In a saucepan over medium heat, add soy milk and stir occasionally until completely melted. Add remaining ingredients and pour into 9 X 13 pan lined with waxed paper. Chill. When firm, cut into pieces.

Granola
4 c. old fashioned oats
2 tsp. cinnamon
2 tsp. vanilla extract
1/3 tsp. stevia
1/4 c. olive oil.
2 Tbsp. rice syrup
Preheat oven to 325 degrees. Mix all ingreidents together and stir until well blended and oats are thoroughly coated with oil. Spread onto a 9 X 13 sheet or edged cookie sheet. Bake for about 30 minutes stirring frequently to promote even browning. Cool and store in an airtight container.

Mixed Berry Bar

10 Tbsp. Instant Protein Soy mix
1 c. Grape Nut Cereal
1 c. Fiber Plan daily crunch
1 c. rolled oats
1 1/2 c. dried fruit (cranberries, raisins or other dried fruit)
1 1/2 tsp. cinnamon
1/2 c. honey
1 tsp. stevia
1/2 c. rice syrup
1/2 c. tofu (Mori-Nu)
1/3 c. orange juice concentrate

Combine protein, cereals, oats, fruits, cinnamon and almonds. Set aside. Bring orange juice and stevia to a boil and remove from heat. Immediately combine stevia, tofu and rest of ingredients. Press into 8 X 8 pan and refrigerate for 45-50 minutes or until firm.

Heavenly (Banana) Pudding

12 3 oz. Mori-Nu lite firm tofu
3.4 c. rice milk
1 tsp. vanilla flavoring
1/8-1/4 tsp. powder stevia (to taste)

Mix above ingredients in blender. This recipe makes a wonderful vanilla pudding. To make a banana pudding, add 1 banana to the above mix. Blend and chill. Stir in the chunks of banana just before serving. Garnish with slivered almonds. Serves 4.

Muffins

3/4 c. rice flour
1 1/4 c. spelt flour
3 Tbsp. honey
3 Tbsp. melted butter
1 c. buttermilk or milk
3 tsp. baking powder
3 tsp. baking soda
1 egg beaten

Bake at 425 degrees for 15-20 minutes.

Oat Muffins
1 c. Quinoa
1 c. oat flour
1 1/3 c. rolled oats
1 tsp. stevia
1 tsp. cinnamon
2 tsp. baking powder
1 tsp. soda
 ½ tsp. salt
1/3 c. wheat germ
½ tsp. nutmeg
½ c. chopped dates
1 c. apple juice
2 eggs, beaten
½ c. english walnuts
¼ c. olive or safflower oil
Bake 425 degrees approximately 18 minutes.

Pineapple Cheesecakes (Rose Moyers)
For those of you who can eat dairy products. This is quick, easy and delicious.

1 cup crushed pineapple, drained
2/3 cup cottage cheese
1 tsp. vanilla
1/32 tsp. stevia
¼ pineapple juice
2 medium eggs
dash salt
Drain pineapple, reserve ¼ cup juice. Brush a bit of olive oil inside of 2 - 10 oz. custard cups. Place ½ of the pineapple in each cup and press down to cover bottom of cup. Combine juice, cheese, eggs, stevia, vanilla and salt in blender. Process until very smooth. Pour ½ of cheese mixture on top of pineapple. Bake at 350 degrees about 30 minutes or until set and firm to touch. Cool and refrigerate. Makes 2 servings.

Pineapple Upside Down Cake
1 c. rice flour
1/c. spelt flour
1 tsp. baking soda
1 tsp. baking powder
1 ½ tsp. powdered stevia
1 ¼ tsp. xanthum gum

Mix together and add:
1 egg
¼ c. olive oil
½ c. oat milk
1 tsp. vanilla
Pour into well oiled 9 X 9 i pan. Spread 1 ½ c. unsweetened crushed pineapple over the top. Bake 350 degrees for 25 minutes or until toothpick comes out clean.

Spice and Nut Cake
1 1/2 c. spelt flour
1 1/2 tsp. stevia
1 1/2 c. unsweetened carob chips
3/4 pkg. tofu (gives a soft texture)
1 c. old fashioned oats
2 eggs
1 tsp. vanilla
2 tsp. baking powder
1 tsp. baking soda
1 1/2 tsp. cinnamon
1/2 c. rice milk
1/2 tsp. found cloves
1/4 tsp. nutmeg
1/2 c. coconut (unsweetened)
½ c. ground english walnuts
Mix together and bake in a 9 X 9 pan at 350 degrees for 20-25 minutes.
Topping:
3/4 c. finely ground walnuts
1/4 c. unsweetened coconuts
melted together:
2 1/2 tsp. butter
2 Tbsp. barley malt syrup
Mix together and spread over cake.

Wonderful Snack-N Cake
1 c. rice flour
1 c. oat flour
1 tsp. soda
1 tsp. baking powder
1 1/2 tsp. powdered stevia
Mix together
In a cup mix together the following:
1 egg
1/4 c. olive oil

1/2 c. soy or oat milk
1 tsp. vanilla
1 1/2 tbsp. rice syrup
Mix together. Add to dry ingredients & mix.
Add the following and stir together:
1/2 c. shredded english walnuts
1/2 c. chopped dates
1/2 c. unsweetened carob chips
Pour into oiled 9X9-inch pan. Bake 375 degrees approximately 20-25 minutes. Great without frosting!

Casseroles

<u>Sweet Onion Tart</u>
1 c. oat flour
2 c. spelt flour
1 tsp. salt
1/4 c. olive oil
3/4 c. butter
2 lbs. of sweet onions
1 large green pepper
1 medium tomato
2 large eggs
1 c. milk 1/2 c. parmesan cheese
1 tsp. chopped thyme
1/2 tsp. cilantro
1 Tbsp. fresh parsley
1/4 c. black pepper
1/4 c. cheddar cheese
Crust: Cut shortening (olive oil and 1/2 c. butter) into flour and salt. Sprinkle in 7-8 Tbsp. cold water until soft enough to form dough. Roll out on flowered surface. Refrigerate about 30 minutes. Melt remaining butter. Add onions and cook until golden. Cool to room temperature. Bake shell at 425 degrees for 20 minutes with weights to hold down shell. Remove weights and bake for 10 more minutes. In bowl beat eggs, milk, cheese, thyme, parsley, pepper and salt. Spread onions in crust. Poor egg mixture over. Bake 25 minutes.

Shrimp and Rice Casserole

1 c. dry rice
2-3 tsp. butter
Sauté till golden brown (about 7 minutes).
3/4 c. onion (chopped)
1 c. diced celery
Add rice and saut`e 3-5 minutes.
4 c. tomato juice
Pinch cayenne or red pepper
1/8 c. parsley flakes
Add and simmer 10-15 minutes.
2 1/2 c. shrimp (about 1 lb.)
2 small cans diced tomatoes
Mix in well. Bake covered for 30 minutes at 350 degrees.

Spinach Casserole

2 packages frozen chopped spinach
2 ½ Tbsp. chopped onion
2 eggs, beaten
1 cup fat free parmesan cheese
8 oz. vegetable sour cream
1 ½ c. spelt or vegetable spaghetti, cooked
Combine above ingredients in a casserole dish. Bake at 350 degrees until bubbly.

Rice Pilaf

1/4 c. butter
1 medium onion
1 medium garlic clove (chopped)
1/2 c. celery
Saute till onion is tender. *Add:*
1/2 c. dry rice
1/4 c. chopped parsley
dash of pepper
1/3 bay leaf
1/8 tsp. thyme
2 1/2 chicken broth
Bring to boil, cover, reduce and simmer 20 minutes +/- rice is done.

Drinks

Egg Nog
5 eggs
24 oz. soft tofu
1 1/2 tsp. vanilla
2 1/2 tsp. nutmeg
3/4 tsp. stevia
1 quart rice milk
2 Tbsp. Shaklee Soy Powder
Blend eggs and tofu in blender. Add remaining ingredients and blend on low.

Ginger Lemon Iced Tea
1/2 c. chopped ginger
2 quarts water
Boil water and ginger for 20 minutes. Let set 2 hours and drain water. *To water add:*
Juice squeezed from 6 lemons
1 to 2 tsp. stevia (sweeten to taste)
Serve over ice.

Meats

"Fishless" Fillets
Freeze 1 pkg. tofu, thaw, and squeeze out excess water with a paper towel. Cut into 6 equal slices.
1-c. bread or cracker crumbs
1 T. parmesan cheese
¼ tsp. garlic salt
¼ tsp. onion powder
¼ tsp. paprika
Baste fillets with olive oil. Roll in mix and bake for 20 minutes at 350 degrees. Serve in a bun as a fish fillet.

Linda's Grey Poupon Marinade for Chicken
1/2 c. olive oil
1/4 c. red win or balsamic vinegar
2 tsp. diced rosemary
1 tsp. minced fresh garlic
2 Tbsp. Grey Poupon
Mix together. Marinate chicken 12 hours or longer. Cut chicken breasts at least in half, tendering with meat tenderizer (wood or metal).

Salmon Kedgeree

1 can (15 1/2 oz.) salmon
1 c. chopped onions
1 clove garlic (minced)
2 tsp. curry powder
3 Tbsp. butter
Chicken broth
1 c. uncooked rice
1/4 tsp. paprika
1/2 c. chopped parsley
Lemon juice

Drain salmon reserving liquid. Break up and set aside. Cook onions, garlic, curry and butter till soft, but not brown. Add enough chicken broth to salmon liquid to equal 2 cups. Add rice in saucepan. Add paprika. Bring to boil, reduce heat, cover and simmer for 20 minutes or until rice is tender and liquid is absorbed. Gently add to salmon 1/3 c. parsley and lemon juice to rice. Cover and heat gently but thoroughly. Garnish with remaining parsley.

Salads

Broccoli Salad

2 bunches broccoli (copped small)
1/2 c. chopped onion
2/3 c. raisins
1/2 c. chopped walnuts (great with black walnuts)
Mix well:
1 c. Nayonnaise
1/3 tsp. stevia
3 Tbsp. vinegar

Best to let sit refrigerated for several hours

Broccoli and Grape Salad

3 c. broccoli (chopped)
1 c. red grapes (halved)
1 chopped onion
7 slices turkey bacon (broken up)
1/3 c. cashews
Dressing
1/2 c. Nayonnaise
1/4 tsp. stevia
1Tbsp. Wine vinegar

Mix dressing ingredients together. Chill broccoli, grapes and onion with dressing for 12 hours. Stir in bacon and cashews before serving.

Carrot Salad

2 c. shredded carrots
½ c. raisins
1/3 c. apple juice
2/3 c. Nayonnaise
Pinch of stevia

Mix together and refrigerate for 2-4 hours before serving.

Curry Chicken Salad

4 ½ c. chopped cooked chicken
¾ c. Nayonnaise (mayonnaise substitute)
½ c. chutney (chopped
1 ½ tsp. cury powder
1 Tbsp. lemon or lime juice
1/12c. toasted almonds

Mix above ingredients and refrigerate before serving. If you cannot find chutney in your grocery store, the following mixture may be used.

(Chutney Mixture)
¼ c. unsweetened, chopped pineapple
1 tsp. apple cider vinegar
1 Tbsp. minced tomato
¼ tsp. paprika
¼ tsp. salt
1/8 tsp. pepper
1 tsp. minced onion
1/16th tsp. powdered stevia

Fruit and Barley Salad

16 oz pearl barley
2 3/4 tsp. salt
4 medium limes
1/3 c. olive oil
1 Tbsp. sugar
3/4 tsp. coursely ground black pepper
1 1/2 lbs. nectarine (4 medium)
1 lb. tomatoes (2 large) cut
4 green onions
1/2 c. chopped fresh mint leaves

Cook barley in salt water. Rinse in cold water. Grate 1 Tbsp. peel of limes and squeeze 1/2 c. juice. Wisk juice, olive oil, sugar, pepper and 1 1/4 tsp. Salt. Add all ingredients. Can be covered and refrigerated.

Honey Mustard Dressing
3/4 c. dijion mustard
1/4 c. sour cream
1/4 c. honey
3/4 tsp. Worcesteshire

Pasta House Salad (Rose Moyers)
1 head iceberg lettuce
1 cup artichoke hearts
1 cup diced pimentos
2/3 cup red wine vinegar
¼ tsp. black pepper
½ head romaine lettuce
1 cup sliced red onion
1/3 cup olive oil
1 tsp. salt
2/3 cup freshly grated parmigiano cheese
Wash the lettuce and drain completely. Place in refrigerator to chill. When it is well chilled, break into small pieces. DO NOT USE A KNIFE ON LETTUCE. Place lettuce into large bowl. Drain artichoke hearts well, measure and add to lettuce. DO NOT USE MARINATED ARTICHOKE HEARTS. Peel and thinly slice red onion. Drain pimentos completely or salad will turn red. Measure the onions and pimentos and add to lettuce. Put oil, vinegar, salt and pepper in jar; shake well. Pour on salad, add Parmigiano cheese and toss until completely mixed. Makes 4 large servings.

Red Bean salad
2 c. cooked red beans
4 hard boiled eggs
½ c. chopped celery
1 cucumber, peeled and chopped
1 sm. clove garlic, chopped
Dressing
1/3 c. Nayonnaise
1/3 c. firm tofu
¼ c. soy or rice milk
½ Tsp. sea salt
1 ¼ tsp. mustard
¼ tsp. dill weed

Mix together and chill before serving.

Spinach Salad
1 bag spinach
7 strips turkey bacon
1 can sliced water chestnuts
4 large mushrooms (sliced)
4 hard-boiled eggs (sliced)
Dressing
1/2 tsp. stevia
1/2 c. catsup
2 tsp. Worcestershire
1 cu. salad oil
1/4 cu. vinegar
2 small cloves garlic
1 chopped onion

Summer Salad
4 cu. semolina macaroni
3 eggs (hard boiled and chopped)
1/2 medium green pepper (chopped)
1/2 medium red pepper (chopped)
1 Tbsp. chopped onion
2 large celery (chopped)
2 cu. cherry tomatoes
1/8 c. chopped fresh parsley
Dressing
3/4 c. fat free Nayonnaise
1/2 cu. rice milk
2 Tbsp. apple cider vinegar
1/8 tsp. stevia

Mix together and pour over vegetables or pasta. Chill. Serves 10.

5 Bean Salad
Mix well:
2/3 tsp. stevia
1/3 c. salad oil
1 Tbsp. dry mustard
1 tsp. black pepper
Add:
2/3 c. vinegar
Drain 1 can each of:
Kidney beans
Green beans
Wax beans

Lima beans
Garbonzo beans
Chop and add:
1 medium onion
3 stalks celery

Best made the day before serving.

Sauces and Dips

Avocado Spread
1 ripe avocado (peeled and mashed)
1/2 c. fat free cream cheese
1/4 c. fat free Nayonnaise
1 Tbsp. fresh squeezed lemon juice

Blend in blender. Use as a spread for rye, rice or other wheat free crackers or breads.

Bean Dip
30 oz. refried beans
1 c. salsa
4 oz. (1 can) diced green chilies

Combine all in deep bowl. Microwave for 5 minutes on high. Mix and serve.

Christmas CranApple Sauce
1 pkg. whole cranberries
15 apples (cooked and peeled)
    Boil cranberries and apples separately.
1/2 lemon
1/2 tsp. stevia (powder)

Pour cranberries in colander until juice drains.

Christmas Cream Cheese
8 oz. fat free cream cheese
2 Tbsp. fat free sour cream
1/4 c. soy milk
1/2 tsp. parley seed
1/4 c. fresh chives
1/4 c. fresh basil

Blend in blender. Use on rice crackers. Is green in color.

Guacamole
2 ripe avocados (pureed)
2 Tbsp. lemon juice
1/2 tsp. Tabasco
1/2 tsp. chili powder
1-2 clove garlic (minced)

Mix and serve.

Hummus
7 cloves garlic
Tahenie paste to taste
1 can garbonzo beans
1/4 c. sesame oil

Blend in blender and serve with corn flats. (Recipe for corn flats can be found on the side of the Masa package the corn flour comes in.)

Parsley Sauce for Steamed Vegetables
1 c. chicken broth
1 egg yolk
1 Tbsp corn starch
1/8 tsp. pepper
!8 tsp nutmeg
1 Tbsp butter
1 Tbsp. dill weed
¼ tsp. salt

Heat broth. Add ¼ c. broth to beaten egg yolk and corn starch. Stir together and pour into broth. Add remaining ingredients and heat until boiling and thickened. Pour over steamed vegetables.

Veggie Alfredo Sauce (Phyllis Woodson)
1/2 cup unsalted navy beans
1/2 cup blanched slivered almonds or cashews
Blend: 1 tbsp sea salt
4 Tbsp. lemon juice
1/4 cup nutritional food yeast
2 Tbsp. corn starch
2 Tbsp. olive oil
1/4 medium raw onion
1/2 tsp. minced garlic
2 cups water
Season to taste - basil, Italian seasoning, etc.
Put all ingredients in blender with the water. Blend thoroughly until smooth. Put in saucepan and heat, add water to desired consistency.

<u>7 Layer Dip</u>
16 oz. refried beans
1 c. (4 oz). Shredded vegetable, cheddar or Monterey Jack
1 can (2 1/4 oz.) sliced ripe olives (drained)
1 medium tomato (chopped)
1 c. guacamole
1 c. sour cream (vegetable or any)
1 c. salsa

In 10-inch glass deep pie plate, spread beans over bottom. Layer remaining ingredients in order listed. Serve with tortilla chips. Serves about 8.

Soups

<u>Cornbread Chile</u>
1 15 oz. can of chili beans
1 15 oz. can of pork and beans
1 Tbsp. chili powder
1 c. cornmeal.
1 c. oat flour
1/8 tsp. stevia
1 tsp. salt
1/8 c. flaxseed (ground)
3/4 tsp. baking soda
2 eggs (well beaten)
1/4 c. vegetable oil.
1 1/2 c. rice or soy milk
Combine chili beans and chili powder in 2-quart casserole dish. Mix the remaining ingredients and pour over bean mixture. Bake at 350 degrees for 45 minutes or until cornbread mixture is lightly brown and done.

<u>Chili</u>
32 oz. bag dried pinto beans (Cover with 1 inch of water.)
2 medium onions
1 clove garlic
2 14 1/2 oz cans stewed tomatoes
1 5 oz. can tomato sauce
2 6 oz. tomato puree
1/2 tsp. black pepper
Cook beans as directed on package. Drain. Add rest of ingredients and simmer 1-2 hours. Leftovers can be frozen for future meals.

Minestrone (Rose Moyers)
1 medium onion, chopped
1 can fat-free beef broth (14 ½ oz.)
1 ½ cups water
2 ½ oz. (1/2 cup) uncooked macaroni
2 tbsps. shredded fresh parmesan cheese
1 tsp. olive oil
1 can Italian recipe tomatoes (14 ½ oz.)
1 ½ cups frozen mixed vegetables
1 can red kidney beans, drained, rinsed
Heat olive oil over medium heat until hot. Add onion; cook until onion is tender. Add broth, tomatoes and water. Bring to a boil. Stir in mixed vegetables, macaroni and kidney beans. Return to a boil. Reduce heat to medium, cook 10 to 15 minutes or until vegetable and macaroni are tender, stirring occasionally. Sprinkle each serving with cheese, if desired. Makes 4 servings.

Split Pea Soup
1 c. dried split peas
2 c. water
Boil for approximately 30 minutes.
Add:
1 medium onion
2 garlic cloves
1 tsp. sea salt
½ tsp. pepper
Simmer for another 15 minutes. Serve hot with rice crackers.

Vegetables

Baked Potatoes
To create a wonderful, yet easy meal, begin with
4 large potatoes that have been scrubbed. Put them into a casserole dish with 3 Tbsp. water. Cover and bake in a 400-degree oven for approximately 1 hour or until soft. Serve the potatoes topped with any of the following toppings:
Barbecue TVP (one of our favorites)
Picante sauce and plain yogurt
Spaghetti sauce
Onions and garlic sautéed in butter and topped with spaghetti sauce.
Tuna salad
Broccoli and goat or vegetable cheese
Baked Beans
Beans of any kind

Creamed Onions

2 pounds onions
¼ cup shredded vegetable cheese
1 Tbsp. butter
3 Tbsp. corn starch
1 cup skim milk
1 tsp. sea salt
½ tsp. pepper

Cook onions in water until done. Melt butter, in saucepan. Add ½ cup of milk. Stir cornstarch into remainder ½ cup of milk and add to melted butter. Add salt and pepper, heating milk and cornstarch mixture, stirring constantly until thickened. Drain onions and add creamed milk. Stir in cheese. Serve.

Delicious Grill

1 onion (cut into large pieces)
4 carrots (cut into 1-inch diagonal pieces)
¼ head cabbage (cut into large pieces)
3 broccoli tops cut up
¼ head of couliflower
2 medium size garlic cloves
½ cup fresh parsley
½ cup fresh lemon thyme (minced)
2 Tbsp. olive oil
Charcoals on grill
Heavy iron skillet

Place iron skillet on coals with oil in it. As soon as skillet is hot put vegetables into it. Put the cover over the grill and let vegetables cook, stirring occasionally to keep from burning. Serve hot.

French Carrots

2 Tbsp. butter (melt and add)
1 1/2 lbs. carrots (cut Julienne)
1/4 tsp. dried basil
1/8 tsp. nutmeg
1/2 c. golden raisins

Cover and cook butter, carrots, basil and nutmeg over low heat about 10 minutes. (May need a little water.) Add raisins, cover and cook 5 minutes or until carrots are tender.

Grilled Potatoes (Rose Moyers)
4 medium to large potatoes
Salt and pepper to taste
2 tbsp. butter
Peel and cut potatoes into ½" cubes. Lightly oil a large piece of heavy-duty aluminum foil and put the potatoes on foil. Salt and pepper and distribute pieces of butter over the potatoes. Tightly wrap (with double folds) the foil over the potatoes and grill on a hot grill until potatoes are tender (about 45 minutes to 1 hour).

Herbed Vegetables
4 long carrots (cleaned & cut into 1 inch pieces)
(Steam 18 minutes)
Meanwhile sauté' in 2 tbsp. butter:
1 medium onion
1 lrg. garlic clove
Add potatoes & carrots to onion mixture.
Mix together:
1 tsp. rosemary
½ tsp. basil
Toss onto potato mixture, serve hot. (4 servings)

Old Fashion Fried Potatoes
2 tbsp. butter
2 garlic cloves
1 med onion
Lightly saute onion and garlic in butter 5 minutes. *Add:*
¾ c. shredded cabbage
2 medium potatoes, (cut in pieces)
Cover and cook until potatoes are tender, stirring occassionally. Salt and pepper to taste.

Veggie Wraps
Lettuce leafs
¼ c. cucumber or green zuchinni
¼ c. onion
alfalfa sprouts
1 guacamole, cut in pieces
feta cheese
poppy seed dressing
Layer vegetables in lettuce leaves. Sprinkle feta cheese over vegetables and drizzle dressing over vegetables. Wrap cabbage roll style. Refrigerate for 2 hours before serving.

Zucchini Boats

Slice zucchini in half lengthwise. Sprinkle with salt, pepper, paprika, onions, fresh garlic and chili powder. Bake in 400 degrees oven until tender. Serve hot.

Misc.

Black Bean Tortilla Pockets (Rose Moyers)
1 can black beans (15 oz.), drained, rinsed
¼ cup chopped green onions
1 tsp. chili powder
1/3 cup tomato sauce (no-salt-added)
4 (8-inch) tortillas
2 oz. shredded cheddar cheese (1/2 cup)
1 medium tomato, chopped
½ tsp. cumin
1 tbsp. lime juice
2 cups shredded lettuce
Combine all ingredients except tortillas and lettuce in medium bowl; mix well. Spoon ¼ of bean mixture evenly down center of each tortilla. Top each with ¼ cup lettuce. Fold bottoms of tortillas up; fold sides toward center, overlapping slightly. Secure with toothpicks. Makes 4 sandwiches.

Refried Beans
16 oz. Dried pinto beans cooked as directed. *Drain and add:*
½ tsp. salt
¾ c. water
Mash. Can be frozen.

Linda's Baked Beans
Low-fat ham (cubed)
4 medium onions (sliced)
Cook together.
1/2 tsp. stevia powder
1/2 c. vinegar
1/4 tsp. dry mustard
Add and simmer 15 minutes.
1 lb. can red beans
1 lb. can butter beans
1 lb. can green limas
2 medium cans pork and beans
Drain and add.
Bake at 350 degrees for 1 hour.

Mexican Sandwich

3/4 can refried beans
2 c. shredded salad greens
1/8 c. shredded carrots
1/2c. light cottage cheese
picante sauce
4 large soft taco shells

Spread beans evenly over soft shells. Divide cottage cheese and carrots and greens over beans. Top with picante sauce and roll. Store in plastic wrap in the refrigerator for up to 24 hours. Makes 4.

Summertime Linguine (Rose Moyers)
This is wonderful, for those of you who aren't allergic to tomatoes!

2 pints cherry tomatoes, halved
¼ cup extra-virgin olive oil
2 tbsp. drained capers
½ tsp. salt
3 tbsp. grated parmesan cheese
1 small red onion, minced
¼ cup ripe olives, quartered
1 tbsp. minced fresh thyme
1 pkg. (16 oz.) linguine (semolina)

In large bowl, combine cherry tomato halves, minced red onion, olive oil, olives, capers, thyme and salt. Cover and chill 2 hours. Cook linguine, drain, and place in large serving bowl. Add tomato mixture to linguine; toss gently to combine. Sprinkle with grated Parmesan cheese. Makes 8 servings.

Quick Turkey Pasta (Rose Moyers)
1 Tbsp. butter
2 garlic cloves, minced
1 Tbsp. cornstarch
½ cup fresh peas
6 green onions, chopped
½ pound turkey breast, cut in strips
1 - 1 ½ cups chicken broth
6 oz. semolina linguini

Sauté onions and garlic in butter until tender. Add turkey breast strips and sauté until just slightly browned. Stir in cornstarch and chicken broth, then peas. Cook until peas are done (just a few minutes). Meanwhile, cook pasta until done. Serve turkey and sauce over pasta.

Stretching Exercises

1. Do not eat at least one hour before stretching (do not start on a full stomach).
2. These exercises are meant to be done very slowly and smoothly. Count to fifteen with each form before changing to a different exercise.
3. Begin taking three deep breaths before starting. Follow these steps for deep breathing: • Sit or stand tall noting the spinal chord being aligned and straight. • Begin to breath in through the nose filing the abdomen area first then the chest area. • Count to seven slowly while breathing in. • Breath out through the mouth to the count of seven, allowing air to leave the belly area first.
4. Slow, deep breaths should be taken during the exercises, exhaling on downward bends, inhaling on upward bends.
5. Each position should be held to a slow count of twenty. Remember the idea is to slowly stretch and strengthen, not to rush through the exercise. It should take approximately twenty minutes for each day's routine.
6. Pain is not the idea of these exercises. The "no pain, no gain" rule does not apply here. Stretch to the point where you feel pulling. Stop and hold that point.
7. Use a soft, relaxing audio tape with either sounds of nature, instrumental music or piano music to keep the atmosphere relaxed. Many audio tapes are twenty minutes long, so they can act as a timer also.
8. Last, enjoy the beauty of the stretches and the flexibility it allows you to have.

Stretching Exercise Plan #1

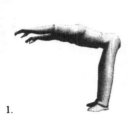 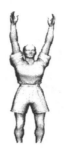 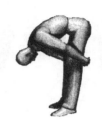

1.   2.   3.

1. Using the back of a chair or wall for support, bend at the waist stretching the back, shoulders and arm muscles. Count to twenty slowly, bend knees and stand up. Repeat this exercise three times.
2. While standing with feet shoulder width apart, move hands above head stretching the back, shoulders and arms. Breathe deeply, then let arms down. Repeat two times.
3. Bend at the waist and grasp hands behind the knees. Pull body close to the legs and hold to a slow count of twenty. Stand up and repeat exercise.

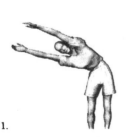 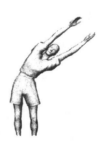 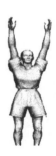

1.   2.   3.

1. With arms above the head as shown in figure #1, bend to the right. Count slowly to twenty.
2. With arms above the head as shown in figure #2, bend to the left, and count slowly to twenty.
3. With arms above the head, stretch the body up into the air as shown in figure #3.
4. Repeat all three exercises two times.

175

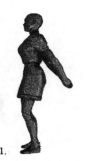
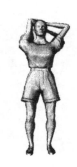
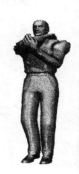

1. 2. 3.

1. While standing up straight, clasp hands behind the back. Breathe in slowly as the arms are lifted as shown in figure #1. Count slowly to twenty to release. Repeat.
2. Place right arm behind the head and with the right hand behind the head, grasp the right elbow with the left hand. Gently stretch the back muscles of the right arms while counting slowly to twenty. Repeat on the opposite side.
3. Bring the right hand over the front of the left shoulder. With the left hand, gently push the right elbow up towards the left shoulder. Hold to a slow count of twenty. Repeat on the opposite side.

Stretching Exercise Plan #2

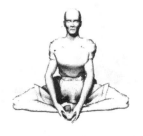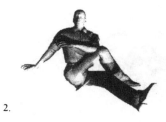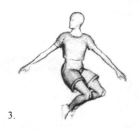

1.

2.

3.

1. While sitting on the floor bring the bottoms of the feet together. Place hands around the feet and gently pull the feet closer to your body. Count slowly to twenty and repeat exercise a second time.
2. Bring the right foot up over the left knee. Put the foot down flat against the floor as shown. Place the right hand on the floor behind you and bring the left hand over to hold the knee firmly. Count slowly to twenty. Repeat on the opposite side.
3. Lie on your back with arms out at the sides and heels against your buttocks. Roll knees over the right side so the left leg is on the floor. Count slowly to twenty and repeat exercise on the left side. Repeat two times.

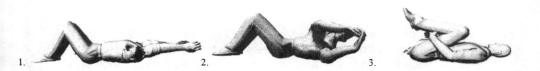

1.

2.

3.

1. Lie on your back with knees bent. Stretch arms above head while breathing deeply. Hold while counting to twenty slowly. Repeat two times.
2. Clasp hands and twist to the right as shown in the figure. Count slowly to twenty. Repeat exercise on opposite side. Repeat complete exercise two times.
3. Lie on your back and bend knees up onto abdomen. Count slowly to twenty. Repeat two times.

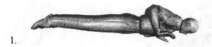 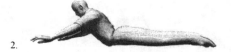

1. Lie on your stomach with forehead on the floor, place hands flat on the floor under shoulders. Count slowly to twenty.
2. With hands still under shoulders push up straightening the arms. Hold this position for a slow count of twenty. Repeat #1 and #2.

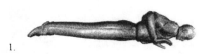 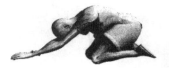

1. Lie on your stomach with forehead on the floor, placing hands flat on the floor under shoulders. Count slowly to twenty.
2. Place feet together and spread knees. With hands together, let the body drop down between the knees stretching arms out in front of the body. Let body relax down to the floor for two to four minutes. Repeat exercises #1 and #2.

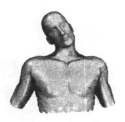 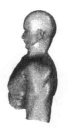 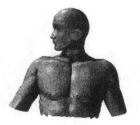 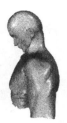

1. While standing or sitting up straight bend the head to the left as if to touch the left ear to the left shoulder. Count slowly to five. Repeat on the right side.
2. Bend the chin towards the neck, as if to make a double chin. Count to five slowly. Turn the head to the right, count slowly to five, then to the left. Count slowly to five.
3. Bend the head forward, then backward, counting slowly to five on each bend.

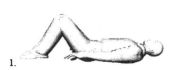 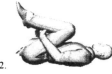 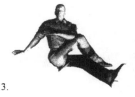

1. While lying on the back, bring the legs up as in figure #1. Count slowly to twenty. Put legs down flat on to the floor. Breathe deeply two times.
2. Bring knees up onto abdomen, grasping hands under the knees. Count slowly to twenty.
3. Bring the right foot up over the left knee. Put the foot down flat against the floor as shown. Place the right hand on the floor behind you and bring the left hand over to hold the knee firmly. Count slowly to twenty. Repeat on the opposite side.

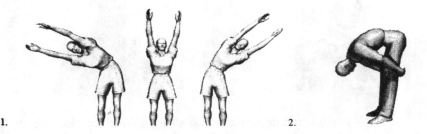

1. With arms above the head as shown, bend to the right. Count slowly to twenty. Move the hands above the head stretching the back, shoulders and arms. Breathe deeply, then let arms down. With arms above the head, bend to the left. Count slowly to twenty. Repeat exercise #1.
2. Bend at the waist and grasp hands behind the knees. Pull body close to the legs and hold to a slow count of twenty. Stand up and repeat exercise #2.

Appendix

TESTING FOR YEAST BYPRODUCTS IN THE URINE OF FIBROMYALGIA PATIENTS

William Shaw Ph.D.

According to William Crook MD, the author of twelve books and numerous medical articles, "CFS/CFIDS and FMS are often yeast related . . . Increasing evidence shows that a sugar-free special diet and anti-fungal medications may help people with these chronic disorders get well." (1). At the Great Plains Laboratory, some of the reasons that yeast overgrowth causes so many problems are becoming clear. Following is a representative report of a urine sample from a patient with severe fibromyalgia. Note that there are four results flagged in the "high or H" category in the yeast/fungal section indicating values that exceed normal limits. The result for tartaric acid is most abnormal. The patient's value is 767 mmol/mol creatinine compared to a normal value of 16 mmol/mol creatinine. (All of these urine values are in terms of urine creatinine to compensate for differences in fluid intake.) Thus, this value for tartaric acid is nearly 50 times that of normal! In addition to the pain of fibromyalgia, this patient complains of depression and unclear thinking.

WHAT IS TARTARIC ACID AND WHAT IS IT DOING IN URINE? The main natural source of tartaric acid is yeast (2). This compound forms a sludge in the wine brewing process and has to be removed (2). Wine is sugar fermented by yeast to alcohol and other products. Humans do not produce this material. When yeast in the intestinal tract are fed sugar from the diet, they produce tartaric acid just like the yeast in the wine-making process. Why is tartaric acid harmful? Tartaric acid is a muscle toxin and as little as 12 grams have been fatal to a human (3). One gram is about the weight of a cigarette.

Tartaric acid is a muscle toxin and caused muscle damage when administered to experimental animals. Tartaric acid is also extremely elevated in many patients with fibromyalgia who also have muscle and joint pain. I initially discovered tartaric acid in the urine of two autistic brothers with muscle weakness so severe that they could not stand up (4).

Tartaric acid is an analog (a close chemical relative) of malic acid (Figure 1). Malic acid is a key intermediate in the Krebs cycle, a biochemical process used for the extraction of most of the energy from our food. Presumably tartaric acid is toxic because it inhibits the biochemical production of the normal compound, malic acid. Tartaric acid is a known inhibitor of the Krebs cycle enzyme fumarase (Figure 2), which produces malic acid from fumaric acid (5). A large percentage of patients with fibromyalgia respond favorably to treatment with malic acid (6). I presume that supplements of malic acid are able to overcome the toxic effects of tartaric acid by supplying deficient malic acid. Treatment with the antifungal drug Nystatin kills the yeast and values for tartaric acid steadily diminish with antifungal treatment (Figure 3). Fifty percent of patients with fibromyalgia often suffer from hypoglycemia (7)(low blood sugar) even though their diet may have adequate or even excessive sugar. The reason may be due to the inhibition of the Krebs cycle by tartaric acid. The Krebs cycle is the main provider of raw material such as malic acid that can be converted to blood sugar (Figure 2) when the body uses up its supply. If sufficient malic acid cannot be produced, the body cannot produce the sugar glucose, which is the main fuel for the brain. The person with hypoglycemia feels weak and their thinking is foggy because there is insufficient fuel for their brain.

WHERE IS THIS YEAST AND WHY DO I HAVE THIS PROBLEM? Most of the time the yeast are present only in the intestinal tract, not in the blood and other organs. However, the tartaric acid and other compounds produced by yeast in the intestine are absorbed into the bloodstream and may enter all of the cells of the body. Dr. St Anand noticed that patients with fibromyalgia had high amounts of dental tartar on their teeth and speculated that similar deposits in the muscles and ligaments might be causing the pain of fibromyalgia. I suspect that tartaric acid is the compound found in the dental tartar and that crystals of this substance may be causing the muscle and joint pain just as kidney stones cause kidney pain. The two main causes of yeast overgrowth are use of broad-spectrum antibiotics and the high sugar and carbohydrate diet of American diet. Broad-spectrum antibiotics kill most of the normal bacteria (germs) in the intestinal tract but do not kill organisms such as yeast (8-15). As a matter of fact, some yeast grows faster in the presence of antibiotics. The reason fibromyalgia commonly follows traumatic accidents may be related to the use of antibiotics to treat trauma. Sugar consumption is the second major factor in causing yeast-related illnesses. The average American consumes 10 times more sugar (about 150 lb. per year) than Americans in the time of George Washington. In a study done in mice, mice receiving sugar in their water had 200 times more yeast in their intestine than mice receiving plain water did (16). Other factors that cause yeast over-growth may include stress, birth control pills, viral infections, and a weak immune system (Figure 4).

WHAT CAN I DO ABOUT THIS PROBLEM IF I HAVE IT? The yeast problem can be treated with a combination of low sugar, low carbohydrate diet, an antifungal drug to kill the yeast, and probiotics, which are supplements of Lactobacillus acidophilus to restore beneficial bacteria to the intestinal tract. Malic acid and magnesium supplements will help the patient until the yeast problem is resolved which may be about two months. The reduction of tartaric acid in urine following antifungal treatment is illustrated in Figure 3.

HOW DO I GET THE TEST DONE? A medical practitioner who is licensed to order urine testing in your state must approve the test order. Regulations vary from state to state so an approved medical practitioner could be a medical doctor (MD), osteopath (DO), nurse practitioner, chiropractor (DC), or naturopath (ND). If you have any difficulty in getting your physician to approve the test, we can refer you to a suitable physician in most locations in the United States and in some foreign countries. The test is reimbursed by most insurance companies but we cannot guarantee reimbursement. A morning urine sample is shipped to The Great Plains Laboratory and results are usually available in 48-72 hours with a recommendation to your physician for treatment.

WHAT OTHER INFORMATION WILL I GET FROM YOUR TEST? The test evaluates all of the well-defined inborn errors of metabolism that can be detected with this technology called GCIMS such as PKU, maple-syrup urine disease, and many others. In addition, I check for many other abnormalities such as vitamin deficiencies and abnormal metabolism of catecholamines, dopamine, and serotonin. We currently quantitate 62 substances but also evaluate other substances that are not quantitated. For example, in the sample report, high kynurenic acid indicated a need for vitamin B-6 and the evaluated glutaric acid indicated a requirement for coenzyme Q10. Even if you don't have the yeast problem, your test may still be beneficial to you.

I HAVE AN HMO AND THEY HAVE TO SEND THE TEST TO A CERTAIN LAB, IS THAT OK? No. No other laboratory routinely analyzes the same compounds as this laboratory including Labcorp, Smithkline, or Mayo Medical laboratories. If you do not specify our laboratory, your urine will be sent to one of the large reference labs, which cannot accurately evaluate your condition. Most test for the inborn errors of metabolism and that's all.

WILL DRUGS OR ANY OF THESE NUTRITIONAL SUPPLEMENTS INTERFERE IN THE ORGANIC ACID TEST? No, there is no interference from any known drug or supplement. However, if antifungal supplements or drugs are taken before the test, you will probably get a lower value for the yeast byproducts. I advise you to get the test first so that you will know what the starting point is. The malic acid and magnesium products will not affect the test results.

I HAVE BEEN DISABLED DUE TO THE SEVERITY OF MY FIBROMYALGIA YET HAVE NOT BEEN ABLE TO GET BENEFITS. COULD THIS TEST HELP ME TO GET BENEFITS? This test could benefit you if we document a defined biochemical disorder. Of greater importance is the possibility of reversing the fibromyalgia if the yeast problem is a significant factor.

WHAT CAN I DO IF MY PHYSICIAN DOESN'T UNDERSTAND THE TEST RESULTS? I will be glad to help you and your physician develop a suitable therapy based on your individual test results.

MY DOCTOR SAYS EVERYONE HAS YEAST IN THEIR INTESTINE AND IF YEAST WERE THE CAUSE OF FIBROMYALGIA THEN EVERY-ONE WOULD BE ADVERSELY AFFECTED. HOW DO ANSWER THAT ASSERTION? The most important question is not whether yeast is present or not. The critical factors are the quantity of yeast and the kinds and amounts of toxic products they produce. Everyone in this society has carbon monoxide in their blood and can tolerate a low value. When the amount of carbon monoxide increases, some individuals feel depressed, some have headaches, some develop muscle weakness, some feel tightness in the chest or angina, some experience nausea and vomiting, some become dizzy, some develop dimming of vision. As values increase, symptoms may include convulsions, coma, respiratory failure, and death. Individuals who recover from severe carbon monoxide poisoning may suffer residual neurological damage. Different people will respond with different symptoms to the same concentration of carbon monoxide. Why is it surprising that exposure to a wide range of toxic yeast products at different times and at different ages might produce different symptoms? If I suggested that there were a carbon monoxide connection with all of the diverse symptoms associated with carbon monoxide exposure, no one would challenge me. The reason that the carbon monoxide connection is accepted is because carbon monoxide can be easily measured in blood. The toxic yeast products were just discovered but as knowledge of them increases, acceptance of the yeast related illnesses would increase. The philosopher Schopenhauer said, "All truth goes through three stages. First, it is ridiculed. Then, it is violently opposed. Finally, it is accepted as self-evident." Within five years, people who ignore the importance of yeast related illness would be in the same camp with those in the Flat-Earth Society.

QUOTED FROM SIDNEY MACDONALD BAKER MD IN THE BOOK DETOXIFICATION AND HEALING, THE KEY TO OPTIMAL HEALTH: "Dr Shaw's work is very recent and as I write this he has just opened a new lab. The reason for telling you about his work is to ask you to think about the implications and watch as his ideas develop over the next few years. As you will see in the next chapter, there is other evidence to support these ideas and, if you understand the implications, there are things you can do now that will reduce your risk of ill health while continuing to watch from the sidelines." Dr. Baker is a graduate of Yale University School of Medicine and is board certified in obstetrics and pediatrics. Dr. Baker was director of the Gessell Institute of Human Development and has taught at Yale Medical School and is the author of dozens of articles and several books about health and nutritional biochemistry.

References

1. Crook William, The Yeast Connection Handbook. Jackson, TN, 1997:34-35.
2. Tartaric acid. Microsoft Encarta 96 Encyclopedia on CD ROM.
3. Webster R. Legal Medicine and Toxicology. WB Saunders, Philadelphia, 1930:413-414.
4. Shaw W. Kassen E, and Chaves E. Increased excretion of analogs of Krebs cycle metabolites and arabinose in two brothers with autistic features. Clinical Chemistry 41:1094-1104,1995.
5. Mahler H and Cordes. Biological Chemistry. New York, Harper and Row. 1966:417-418.
6. Holzschlag Molly. CoQ1O, malic acid, and magnesium may improve CFIDSIFM symptoms. The CFIDS Chronicle, Summer 1993.
7. St Amand RP. Exploring the fib romyalgia connection. The Vulvar Pain Newslet-ter. Fall 1996,4-6.
8. Kennedy M and Volz P Dissemination of yeasts after gastrointestinal inoculation in antibiotic-treated mice. Sabouradia 21:27-33,1983.
9. Danna P, Urban C, Bellin E, and Rahal J. Role of Candida in pathogenesis of antibiotic associated diarrhoea in elderly patients. Lancet 337:511-14, 1991.
10. Osfleld E, Rubinstein E, Gazit E, Smetana Z. Effect of systemic antibiotics on the microbial flora of the extemal ear canal in hospitalized children. Pediat 60:364-66,1977. 11. Kinsman OS, Pitblado K. Cand ida albicans gastrointestinal colonization and invasion in the mouse: effect of antibacterial dosing, antifungal therapy, and immunosuppression. Mycoses 32:664-74, 1989.
12. Van der Waaij D. Colonization resistance of the digestive tract-mechanism and clinical consequences. Nahrung 31:507-17,1987.
13. Samonis G and Dassiou M. Antibiotics affecting gastrointestinal colonization of mice by yeasts. Chemotherapy 6: 50-2,1994.
14. Samonis G., Gikas A, and Toloudis, P. Prospective evaluation of the impact of broad-spectrum antibiotics on the yeast flora of the human gut. Euro Jour of Clin Micro Infec Dis, 13(1994): 665-67.
15. Samonis G, Gikas A, and Anaissie E. Prospective evaluation of the impact of broad-spectrum antibiotics on gastrointestinal yeast colonization of humans. Antimicrobian agents and Chemotherapy 37(1993): 51-53.
16. Vargas S, Patrick C, Ayers G, and Hughes W. Modulating effect of dietary carbohydrate supplementation on Candida albicans colonization and invasion in a neutropenic mouse model. Infection and Immunity 61(1993): 619-626.

THE GREAT PLAINS LABORATORY

9335 W. 75 St.
Overland Park, KS 66204

Phone (913) 341-8949
Fax   (913) 341-6207

CLIA ID# 17D0919496
William Shaw Ph.D., Laboratory Director

Patient Name	Jane Doe	Date of collection	2/11/97
Patient Age	36	Time of collection	8:50 AM
Physician Name	John Smith, MD	Patient Sex	Female

Name	mmol/mol creatinine		Reference range mmol/mol creatinine	Name	mmol/mol creatinine		Reference range mmol/mol creatinine
Glycolysis				**Yeast/Fungal**			
lactic	22.15		0-100	citramalic	4.42	H	0-2
pyruvic	9.82		0-50	5-hydroxymethyl-2-furoic	98	H	0-80
2-hydroxybutyric	1.06		0-2	3-oxoglutaric	0.46		0-0.5
glyceric	8.17		0-10	furan-2,5-dicarboxylic	67.01	H	0-50
Amino Acid Metabolites				furancarbonylglycine	0		0-60
2-hydroxyisovaleric	0.10		0-2	tartaric	767	H	0-16
2-oxoisovaleric	0.19		0-2	arabinose	27		0-115
3-methyl-2-oxovaleric	0.24		0-2	carboxycitric	0.81		0-46
hydroxyisocaproic	0.02		0-2	**Bacterial**			
2-oxoisocaproic	0.23		0-2	2-hydroxyphenylacetic	0.61		0-10
2-oxo-4-methiolbutyric	0.03		0-2	4-hydroxyphenylacetic	41		0-50
mandelic	0.31		0-5	**Anaerobic Bacterial**			
phenyllactic	0.24		0-2	DHPPA analog	103		0-150
phenylpyruvic	0.14		0-5	VMA analog	15.41		0-31
homogentisic	0.87		0-2	**Krebs Cycle**			
4-hydroxyphenyllactic	2		0-50	succinic	3		0-20
pyroglutamic	9	L	20-115	fumaric	1.31		0-10
3-indoleacetic	8.68		0-10	2-oxo-glutaric	29.57		15-200
kynurenic	2.82	H	0-2	aconitic	35	H	0-25
Fatty Acid Metabolites				citric	23		20-200
3-hydroxybutyric	0.78		0-10	**Neurotransmitters**			
acetoacetic	17.12	H	0-10	HVA	16.53		0-25
ethylmalonic	0.08		0-10	VMA	3.23		0-18
methylsuccinic	2.68		0-5	5-hydroxyindoleacetic	1.08		0-20
adipic	6.41		0-12	**Pyrimidines**			
suberic	3.67	H	0-2	uracil	11.96		0-22
sebacic	1.28		0-2	thymine	0.33		0-2
Miscellaneous				**Miscellaneous**			
glutaric	2.21	H	0-2	glycolic	57		0-100
methylmalonic	1.09		0-5	oxalic	17.06		0-100
N-acetyl aspartic	8.44		0-100	malonic	0.20		0-10
ascorbic	8501.43	H	10-200	methylglutaric	0.89		0-10
orotic	0.06		0-3.5	hippuric	677	H	10-400
3-hydroxy-3-methylglutaric	3.31		0-36	4-hydroxybutyric	2.34		0-5
hydroxyhippuric	2.08		0-20	phenylcarboxylic	0.21		0-15
				indole-like compound	9.56		0-60

Figure 1. Comparison of chemical structure of malic and tartaric acid. Differences are shaded in gray.

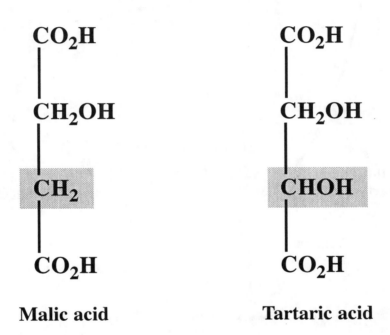

Malic acid   Tartaric acid

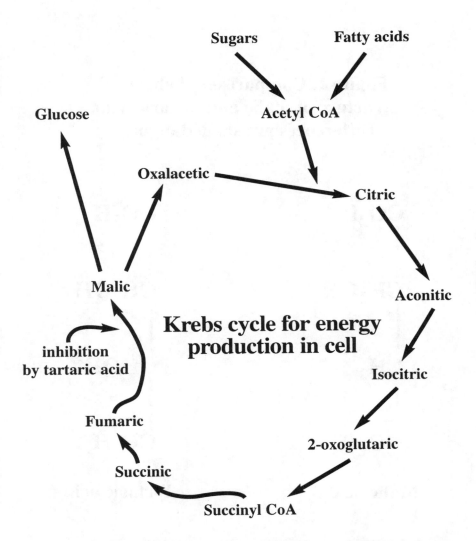

**Figure 2. Site of tartaric acid inhibition of Krebs cycle,
the major energy producing mechanism of the cell. In
addition to the inhibition of energy production, tartaric
acid prevents the production of malic acid which is a key
intermediate in the production of glucose in the process
of gluconeogenesis, the principal fuel for the brain.**

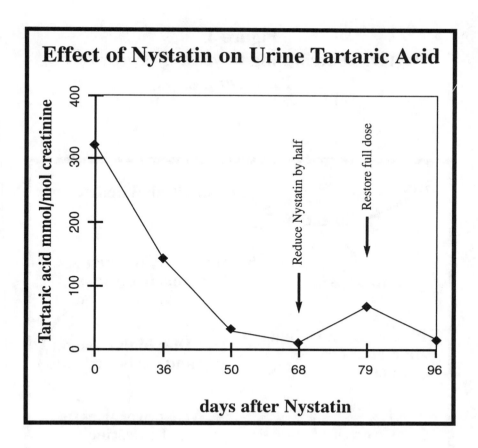

Figure 3. Patient with high tartaric acid was started on the antifungal drug Nystatin and then tested while on this drug. Even after 68 days tartaric increased when the dose was reduced in half and then decreased again when the full dose of antifungal drug was restored.

Figure 4.
Factors contributing to yeast overgrowth in fibromyalgia.

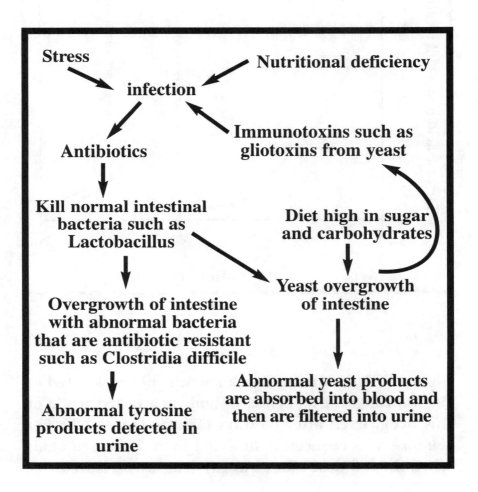

RESOURCES

Fibromyalgia Solutions
305 E. 9th Street
Kearney, MO 64060
816-903-5427
www.fibrosolutions.com

Nebraska Natural Medical Center
7643 Cass Street
Omaha, NE 68114
402-399-2020

Dr. David Yoo
153 W. 151st Street
Ste. 150
Olathe, KS 66061
913-393-0150

Sastun Center of Integrative
   Health Care
5509 Foxridge Drive
Mission, KS 66202
913-384-2284

Dr. Varsha Rathod
138 N. Merimec
Clayton, MO 63105
314-721-7227

Family Chiropractic Clinic
110 NE Trilein
Ankeny, IA 50021
515-965-1810

St. Luke's Center for Health
   And Well-Being
810 First Avenue NE
PO Box 3026
Cedar Rapids, Iowa 52406-3026
319-369-8161

Dr. Pavel Yutsis
Yutsis Center for Integrative
   Medicine
6413 Bay Parkway
Brooklyn, NY 11204
718-621-0900

Great Plains Laboratory
11813 W. 77th St.
Lenexa, KS 66214
913-341-8949
www.greatplainslaboratory.com

Dr. Carol Ann Ryser
5308 E. 115th Street
Kansas City, MO 64137-2731
816-763-9165

American Academy of Medical
   Acupuncture
5820 Wilshire Blvd., Suite 500
Los Angeles, CA 90036
213-937-5541
www.medicalacupuncture.org

American Association of
   Alternative Medicine, Inc.
1000 Rutherford Road
Landrum, SC 29356

American Association of
   Naturopathic Physicians
601 Valley Street, Suite 105
Seattle, WA 98109
206-298-0126

American Association of Oriental
   Medicine
433 Front Street
Catasauqua, PA 18032
610-266-1433

American Holistic Medical
   Association
6728 Old McLean Village Drive
McLean, VA 22101
703-556-9728

Fibromyalgia Coalition International
PO Box 9509
Mission, KS 66201-1509
913-384-4673

Mail Order Catalog for
   Healthy Living
P.O. Box 180
Summertown, TN 38483
800-695-2241

Bibliography

Chevallier, A. (1996). The Encyclopedia of Medicinal Plants. New York, NY: DK Publishing, Inc.

Crook, W.G. (1995). Chronic Fatigue Syndrome and the Yeast Connection. Jackson, TN: Professional Books.

Crook, W. G. (2001). Tired-So Tired and the "Yeast Connection." Jackson, TN: Professional Books.

Edgson, V., & Marber, M. (1999). The Food Doctor: Healing foods for the mind and body. New York, NY: Collins & Brown.

Elrod, J.M. (1997). Reversing Fibromyalgia. Pleasant Grove, UT: Woodland Publishing.

Gach, M.R. (1990). Acupressure's Potent Points. New York, NY: Bantam Books.

Kellas, W.R., & Dworkin, A.S. (1996). Thriving in a ToxicWorld. Olivenhain, CA: Professional Preference.

Lad, V. (1998). The Complete Book of Ayurvedic Home Remedies. New York, NY: Harmony Books.

Monte, T. (1997). The Complete Guide to Natural Living. New York, NY: Perigee.

Nightingale, M. (1987). Acupuncture. Rutland, VT: Charles E. Tuttle Company, Inc.

Ody, P. (1993). The Complete Medicinal Herbal. London: Dorling Kindersley.

Somer, E. (1992). The Essential Guide to Vitamins and Minerals. New York, NY: HarperPerennial, a Division of HarperCollins Publishers.

Teitelbaum, J. (1996). From Fatigued to Fantastic. Garden City Park, NY: Avery Publishing Group.

Time Life Editors. (1997). The Alternate Advisor. Alexandria, VA: Time Life Books.

Wallach, J.D., & Lan, M. (1989). Let's Play Doctor. Bonita, CA: Double Happiness Publishing Co

CONTACTING MARY

To contact Mary regarding speaking engagements or
to order her audiotapes visit her website at
www.fibrosolutions.com or call 888-743-4276.
You can also write Mary at:

Fibromyalgia Solutions
305 East 9th Street
Kearney, MO 64060